Laboratory Manual for
CIVIL
ENGINEERING

SECOND EDITION

Laboratory Manual for
CIVIL ENGINEERING
SECOND EDITION

H.S. MOONDRA
RAJIV GUPTA

Birla Institute of Technology & Science,
Pilani (Raj.)

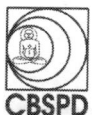

CBSPD

CBS Publishers & Distributors Pvt Ltd

New Delhi • Bengaluru • Chennai • Kochi • Kolkata • Lucknow • Mumbai
Hyderabad • Jharkhand • Nagpur • Patna • Pune • Uttarakhand

Laboratory Manual for
**CIVIL
ENGINEERING**

ISBN: 978-81-239-0150-3

First Edition: 1992
Second Edition: 2000
Reprint: 2009, 2010, 2011, 2012, 2013, 2014, 2015, 2019, 2023

Published by **Satish Kumar Jain** and produced by **Varun Jain** for

CBS Publishers & Distributors Pvt Ltd
4819/XI Prahlad Street, 24 Ansari Road, Daryaganj, New Delhi 110 002, India.
Ph: 011-23289259, 23266861   Website: www.cbspd.com
                                    e-mail: delhi@cbspd.com

Corporate Office: 204 FIE, Industrial Area, Patparganj, Delhi 110 092

Ph: 011-4934 4934   Fax: 011-4934 4935   e-mail: publishing@cbspd.com; publicity@cbspd.com

Branches

- **Bengaluru:** Seema House 2975, 17th Cross, KR Road, Banasankari 2nd Stage, Bengaluru 560 070, Karnataka, India
  Ph: +91-80-26771678/79   Fax: +91-80-26771680   e-mail: bangalore@cbspd.com
- **Chennai:** 7, Subbaraya Street, Shenoy Nagar, Chennai 600 030, Tamil Nadu, India
  Ph: +91-44-26680620, 26681266   Fax: +91-44-42032115   e-mail: chennai@cbspd.com
- **Kochi:** 42/1325, 1326, Power House Road, Opp KSEB, Power House, Ernakulum Kochi 682 018, Kerala, India
  Ph: +91-484-4059061-65,67   Fax: +91-484-4059065   e-mail: kochi@cbspd.com
- **Kolkata:** 147, Hind Ceramics Compound, 1st Floor, Nilgunj Road, Belghoria, Kolkata-700056, West Bengal, India
  Ph: +033-25633055, 033-25633056   e-mail: kolkata@cbspd.com
- **Lucknow:** Basement, Khushnuma Complex, 7 Meerabai Marg (Behind Jawahar Bhawan),Lucknow-226001, UP, India
  Ph: +0522-4000032   e-mail: tiwari.lucknow@cbspd.com
- **Mumbai:** PWD Shed, Gala no 25/26, Ramchandra Bhatt Marg, Next to JJ Hospital Gate no. 2, Opp. Union Bank of India, Noorbaug, Mumbai-400009, Maharashtra, India
  Ph: 022-66661880/89   e-mail: mumbai@cbspd.com

Representatives

• Hyderabad	0-9885175004	• Jharkhand	0-9811541605	• Nagpur	0-9421945513
• Patna	0-9334159340	• Pune	0-9923910676	• Uttarakhand	0-9716462459

Printed at Sanjay Printer, Sahibabad, UP, India

PREFACE

A comprehensive Laboratory Manual for Civil Engineering containing the optimum number and type of experiments for an undergraduate curriculum is of much importance to provide the students with requisite knowledge, skills and experience. At present there is a dearth of such manuals that cover the experiments for the different fields of civil engineering that are studied at the undergraduate level in a relevant and comprehensive manner. The manuals currently available deal with specific fields individually and contain a very large number of experiments many of which are of much higher levels than can be possibly considered at the undergraduate stage. A need is thus felt for a laboratory manual which would contain a well selected number of experiments for each of these fields that would provide an appropriate insight into each of them as well as a broad overview of the entire field of civil engineering. The present work is a trial to develop such a manual which aims to equip the students with those aspects which they definitely ought to learn and enable the handling of experiments in a manner that would benefit them most.

Our project had continued support and encouragement from Dr. S. Venkateswaran, Director B.I.T.S., Pilani and we wish to express our heartfelt thanks to him.

We wish to express our thanks to our colleagues Dr. C.L. Dhar, Dr. P.C. Pandey, Dr. D.S.P. Rao for their contribution and continuous encouragement.

Special thanks are due to Dr. S. Ghoshal and the faculty of Civil Engineering group for their help and support.

Needless to say that comments, corrections and constructive criticism are sincerely invited from all the users of this manual and they are thanked in anticipation for the same.

BITS, Pilani (Raj.)

H.S. MOONDRA
RAJIV GUPTA

CONTENTS

SECTION 3

Hydraulic Engineering Laboratory

SECTION 4

Highway Engineering Laboratory

Concrete Laboratory

Structural Engineering Laboratory

Additions to the Second Edition

INTRODUCTION

A laboratory manual for the civil engineering experiments at the under graduate level must provide the students with the requisite insight and skills concerned with the various fields that are studied. The manuals are usually developed to deal with individual fields and there is thus a requirement for a comprehensive manual that encompasses the ones of prime importance under one cover.

The manual deals with the various fields including soil mechanics laboratory, surveying, highway, hydraulic engineering, concrete, structural and public health engineering laboratory.

The first step involves the collection of data and information. Various colleges and universities across the country were requested to provide information regarding the experiments followed there as well as their opinions as regards which of the experiments ought to be included in the curriculum. Based on the analysis that followed the collection of information and diverse opinions from various institutions, it was concluded that a number of 75 experiments chosen with care from different fields would serve as the optimum requirement.

Having identified the nature and aim of the experiments to be included, the methodology for them was prepared. This included

(i)   the apparatus, equipments needed,

(ii) defining the theoretical background and

(iii) procedure for performing the experiment, etc.

Each experiment naturally involves observations, calculations and conclusions, but the manual being prepared includes the limitations of the experiment, precautions to be followed and few suggested questions dealing with the text. The outline of limitations would enable the students to learn the conditions under which the experiment can be performed. Through the questions the students would be able to assess themselves what they have learnt as well as it would facilitate the task of the examiner. Precautions would enable the performer of the experiment in a standard manner to get accurate observations and results.

Many experiments involves lengthy computational work requiring much time. Computer programs in PASCAL have been written which are user friendly, greatly simplifying the task of the students. They only need to feed in their observations and the results would be provided in analytical form.

The various factors that have been taken into consideration while preparing the report are as under :

(i) *Through coverage of the theoretical aspect :*   It was kept in mind that the student who is performing the experiment must know all about the experiment, its physical significance, practical use and the theoretical aspect associated with the experiment. While examining the cross section of students through informal discussion, it was revealed that students know very little about the theoretical and practical consideration of experiment. Though they knew about the procedure and methods adopted in performing the experiments but their basic knowledge in the theoretical matter was very little. To overcome such situation, stress is given in experiments on the theoretical background of the subject which would be of much help to students.

(ii) *Standard Methods :*   In all the experiments it has been decided that the procedure adopted and the methodology presented to perform the experiment should be standard. The method which is widely used is given priority. Wherever the Indian Standard procedure is different from the prevalent method, the salient features of both the methods are also listed in the experiment and a recommendation is made, as to which method is more appropriate to the concerned experiment. This would help student or the experiment performer to know well about the method before conducting the experiment as to which method he should adopt to get the correct results.

(iii) *Laboratory Discipline :* Laboratory equipments are usually quite costly. Careless handling of the equipment results in gross experimental errors. It was borne in mind to train and educate the student in laboratory discipline and a guide line has been presented regarding the handling of the equipments. To save the time, precautions regarding the experiment are also listed. This list of precautions would help student to complete the required task without any difficulty in operating the equipment.

(iv) *Suggested Questions :* Few questions regarding the experiment are also given in this laboratory manual report. This is presented mainly to help the student assess his understanding in that particular experiment. These questions would also provide student a clear picture about the things he has learnt through the experiment and will also help instructor to assess students understanding in that experiment. Questions presented are not straight forward but required an intelligent thought about the subject matter and at the same time the questions are also not very tough and falls within the range of under graduate level.

The report has excluded certain very sophisticated experiments requiring expensive equipments and facilities which are not usually available in all the colleges and institutions. Alternate and simpler methods covering the basic ideas of these experiments have been, however, included in the manual.

This laboratory manual section provides information of a general reference nature. Included in this section are information on laboratory procedures the student is expected to use and a guide to the preparation of laboratory reports which the student may find useful, and also definition as well as volumetric and gravitimetric relationship on all the topics of the civil engineering are covered under the study of this manual. The student should carefully read this section of the manual and refer to it often to ensure correct report form and for methods of preparing graphs to present test information which requires curve plotting.

The following assumptions have been made in general for the experiments to follow in this manual :

1. Soil has weight.
2. Air has no weight.
3. Water has weight. Generally we shall take this as 1 g/cc.

Laboratory Procedure

Laboratory equipment is expensive. Equipment may be damaged by careless handling and damaged equipment may yield serious test errors. Scales are especially susceptible to damage. For this reason, they are not to be moved to other laboratory locations. Before taking any weighing, balances should be checked for zero reading and any aeries of weighing should be taken on the same balance to avoid zero errors between two balances.

The drying ovens are preset to a temperature of 105 to 110 degree Celsius, and the thermostat should not be manipulated without any proper cause as it takes considerable time to stabilize the oven temperature so that the thermostat can be set properly. Oven dried samples should be removed from the oven no later than 24 hours after placing the samples in the oven.

Laboratory Reports

A laboratory report is required for all experiments unless otherwise stated by the instructor. The report should be in a folder on which the following information must be shown :

1. Name of student,
2. Title of experiment,
3. Course number and laboratory section and
4. Date of project and date of report submission.

The report should consist the following information in the given sequence :

1. Flyleaf — showing title of project, name of student, course number, date of work, date of submission of report.

2. Introduction — a brief summary of the objectives of the work.

3. Discussion of the work — including any special techniques used or changes in laboratory manual instructions. Any equipment limitations or possible sources of error should be discussed. If any equations other then basic definitions are used, then include the equations and note that their derivations are shown in the sample calculations. If results are not very good, give analysis of the probable cause.

4. Conclusions — a brief summary and tabulation of the results. If any improvements can be made, these should be listed under this heading. Do not say you got a lot (or nothing) out of the experiment, as this is not considered a 'conclusion'. Be sure to tabulate the test results in this section of the report.

5. Show any graphs next and follow these with the collected data. Do not overwrite on data — get in habit of taking neat laboratory notes.

6. Sample calculations — it is not necessary to show every calculation, but one calculation which is typical should be shown. Be sure to show any derivation required to obtain equations for use in the data reduction.

The report should follow good technical report writing form, including the citing of any references used. Use of first person in writing a technical report should be avoided. Use of such statements as "I found that..." or "My group found..." are generally discouraged. Try to use good sentence construction, and do not change from past to present tense in the same sentence or paragraph.

A primary purpose of the report is to give the instructor an indication of what you learned from the project.

Drawing Graphs

A curve should be legible, and easily understood. It is usually undesirable to paste several semilog paper together to obtain the required number of cycles because of the resulting page folds when the report is bound. The use of graph paper in centimeter divisions is encouraged.

When drawing the curves, always place them on the graph sheet so that the left and the lower margins are both at least 2 cm. wide. All lettering on the axes must be on the ruled portion of the sheet, and the line ruling should be used as lettering guidelines. Use as large a scale as possible, but one which is easy to plot and/or read.

A title block must be shown on all graphs which includes :

1. Title of project

2. Date of work

3. Scale

Always draw smooth curves through plotted points using a french curve. Before plotting graphs, thought must be given to what information the graph is to present. Is it qualitative or quantitative or both? Quantitative information requires a better scale than qualitative information. As an example, plotting a curve which is asymptotic generally displays better with the asymptote horizontal rather than vertical.

The values to be obtained from the plot of experimental data should always be shown on the graph. If these values are used to compute a constant, show both the computation and the constant on the graph.

Laboratory Practice

The procedure outlined in the experiments to follow are reasonably standard. Wherever the Indian Standard Method is available to perform the experiment, it is given as a standard method, but if other methods are also available then those are also given in the experiments.

Soil is highly variable in nature, and this variability cannot be controlled to any great extent. It may be possible to alter its structure or change its composition by mixing it with imported materials. Soil tests are for the purpose of identifying the material, determining certain physical properties of the material, and establishing control criteria for the material.

Since it is obviously impossible to test the entire soil mass and since soil is a variable quantity., it is necessary to perform a few tests on small quantities of soil and extrapolate the results to the entire soil mass.

When using the data sheets, always insert the units of the dial gauges, load rings etc. or any other information which may be needed to complete the test.

LABORATORY EXPERIMENTS

SECTION 1

SOIL MECHANICS LABORATORY

In the soil mechanics laboratory, the properties of soil are determined. The experiment related to some important properties are given in this chapter. The importance of these experiments in civil engineering is as follows :

Atterberg limit gives the idea about the plasticity and the toughness of the soil. The specific gravity of the soil is related with the permeability of soil. A soil is more permeable means that the water can percolate through this soil more easily and at high speed. So the soil underneath the huge structure should not be permeable otherwise piping may occur and the whole structure may collapse. Grain size distribution tells about the size and percentage of particle from which the parent material of soil can be revealed easily and hence it can be classified. Compaction test is very important test. With the help of this test the maximum dry density and optimum water content of the soil can be determined. These results are useful in highway constructions also. Generally the soil subgrade which would be underneath the pavement is compacted at optimum water content to achieve maximum dry density to bear maximum traffic load. Consolidation test is used in determining consolidation properties of the soil.

If soil under steady load settles more than the allowable or the expected value then the structure above the soil may collapse. Therefore before construction of any structure the consolidation properties should be determined properly.

Shearing strength of the soil is the property which resist the lateral pressure and is determined by the shear test. Shearing strength of the soil is considered in the design of an embankment and piers and plays a very important role in designing different type of foundations.

To determine the bearing strength of the soil cone bearing test is performed. Thickness of soil subgrade layer in highway or railway alignment is decided by bearing strength of the soil.

Similar to other properties the compressive strength of the soil is also very important property. It is considered where compressive loads are acting.

Experiment No. 1

Object :

Determination of field density of soil by various methods :
   (i)   Core cutter method
   (ii) Sand replacement method.

A. Core Cutter Method :

Apparatus/Equipment :

Core cutter, rammer, knife, balance, container for water content determination, etc.

Theoretical background :

The weight of soil in core cutter when divided by the volume of core cutter gives the density of soil in situ. The soil in the core cutter is as dense as it is in situ since soil pattern is not disturbed in any way. Hence the density of soil in core cutter can be regarded as the density of soil in situ.

Procedure :

   1. Measure the inside diameter of core cutter and weigh the core cutter.
   2. Choose small area about 30 cm. square and level it. Put the dolly on the top of the core cutter and drive the assembly into the soil until the top of dolly protrudes about 1.5 cm. above the surface.
   3. Dig out the cutter from soil. With the help of straight edge trim flat the end of the cutter. Remove the dolly and trim flat the other end also.
   4. Weigh the cutter full of soil.
   5. Keep some representative soil in oven for 24 hours for water content determination.
   6. Repeat the test at two or three nearby locations and get the average wet and dry density.

Observations :

	Determination No.	1	2	3
1.	Wt. of core cutter			
2.	Wt. of core cutter + soil			
3.	Wt. of wet soil			
4.	Volume of core cutter			
5.	Container No.			
6.	Wt. of container			
7.	Wt. of container + wet soil			
8.	Wt. of container + dry soil			
9.	Wt. of water = (7) − (8)			

Calculations :

		1	2	3
1.	Bulk density $= \dfrac{\text{wt. of soil in core cutter}}{\text{vol. of core cutter}}$			
2.	Water content $= \dfrac{\text{wt. of water}}{\text{wt. of dry soil}}$			
3.	Dry density $= \dfrac{\text{bulk density}}{1 + \text{water content}}$			

Average bulk density =

Average dry density =

Results :

   i) Bulk density = _____

   ii) Dry density = _____

B. Sand Replacement Method :

Apparatus/Equipment :

Sand replacement bottle, water content determination container, balance, tools for excavating, etc.

Theoretical background :

The excavated soil is weighed on balance and its volume is determined indirectly by sand of known bulk density. Thus the field density of soil is determined.

Procedure :

1. Fill the sand in sand replacement bottle (sand pouring cylinder) upto the top and weigh it.
2. Put the cylinder on glass plate and open the shutter, allow the sand to run out. Shut the shutter when there is no further movement of sand. Weigh the sand collected on glass plate. It will give the weight of sand filling the pouring cone.
3. Take a calibrating container and determine its volume by filling it with water, since density of water is known.
4. Fill up the calibrating container by sand (of sand replacement bottle) by placing the bottle on top of container and allowing sand to run into container. Determine the weight of sand filling container and cone.
5. Choose some area about 45 cm square and level it. Place the tray on level surface and excavate a hole of 10 cm diameter and 5 cm depth approximately. Weigh the excavated soil and put some representative of soil in oven for water content determination.
6. Remove the tray and place the sand replacement bottle there open the shutter and allow the sand to run into hole. Close the shutter when no further movement is there in sand. Determine the weight of sand filling hole and cone.

Observations :

1. Wt. of sand in pouring cone = _____
2. Vol. of calibrating container = _____
3. Wt. of sand in calibrating container + cone = _____
4. Wt. of excavated wet soil = _____
5. Wt. of container (water content determination) = _____
6. Wt. of container + wet soil = _____
7. Wt. of container + dry soil = _____
8. Wt. of dry soil = (6) – (7) = _____
9. Wt. of sand in excavated hole and cone = _____

Calculations :

1. Wt. of sand in calibrating container = (3) – (1)

2. Density of sand $= \dfrac{\text{wt. of sand in calibrating container}}{\text{vol. of calibrating container}}$

3. Wt. of sand in excavated hole =

4. Vol. of hole $= \dfrac{\text{wt. of sand in excavated hole}}{\text{density of sand}}$

5. Bulk density of soil $= \dfrac{\text{wt. of excavated soil}}{\text{vol. of hole}}$

6. Water content $= \dfrac{\text{wt. of water}}{\text{wt. of dry soil}}$

7. Dry density of soil $= \dfrac{\text{bulk density of soil}}{1 + \text{water content}}$

Results :

    i) Bulk density = _____

   ii) Dry density = _____

Questions :

    1. Compare the results obtained from the two methods.

    2. Which method is best suited for determination of field density?

    3. Define dry, wet and saturated densities of the soil.

    4. What do you understand by submerged density?

    5. Mention the field conditions under which different types of densities have to be used.

    6. Out of these various type of densities, which one of them is maximum and minimum? Explain.

Experiment No. 2

Object :

(a) To determine the specific gravity of soil by pycnometer.

(b) To determine the water content of a soil sample whose specific gravity (sp. gr. of soil solids) by pycnometer is known and check it with oven drying method.

a. Determination of specific gravity :

Apparatus/Equipment :

A pycnometer (fitted with a conical brass cap screwed at its top), balance (sensitive to 1 gm), glass rod or some stirrer, oven.

Theoretical background :

The specific gravity G of the soil solids is the ratio of the unit weight of soil solids to that of water at a given temperature.

$$G = \frac{\rho_s}{\rho_w}$$

ρ_s = unit wt. of soil solid

ρ_w = unit wt. of water

Unit weight is defined as weight per unit volume.

Procedure :

1. Weigh the dry and empty pycnometer. Let this be W_1.
2. Take about 200 gm oven dried soil and put it in pycnometer. The pycnometer and sand (W_2).
3. Add some water in it and mix it thoroughly with glass rod. Add some more water and stir it. Fill the pycnometer by water upto the hole of conical cap, dry the pycnometer from outside and weigh it (W_3).
4. Empty the pycnometer, clean it thoroughly and fill it with distilled water to the hole of conical cap and weigh it (W_4).
5. Repeat the steps from 2 to 4 for two or three readings and find the average specific gravity.

Observations :

		1	2	3
1.	Wt. of pycnometer (W_1 gm)			
2.	Wt. of pyc + dry soil (W_2 gm)			
3.	Wt. of pyc + soil + water (W_3 gm)			
4.	Wt. of pyc + water (W_4 gm)			
5.	Sp. gravity			
6.	Av. sp. gravity			

Result :

The average specific gravity =

b. Determination of water content :

Theoretical background :

The water content of any soil sample can be determined by pycnometer if soil solid specific gravity (G) is known.

Derivation :

Wt. of water + pyc (W_4) $= W_3 - W_d + \dfrac{W_d}{G}$

W_d = wt. of solid particles

$\dfrac{W_d}{G}$ = volume of solid particles and also the weight of water of volume $\dfrac{W_d}{G}$ (since $\rho_w = 1$ in C.G.S.)

$\left(\dfrac{G-1}{G}\right) W_d = W_3 - W_4$

$W_d = \dfrac{W_3 - W_4}{G - 1} \times G$

Wt. of soil sample $= W_2 - W_1$

Wt. of water in soil sample $= W_2 - W_1 - W_d$

Water content $w = \dfrac{W_w}{W_d} \times 100$

$= \dfrac{\left(-\dfrac{W_3 - W_4}{G - 1} \times G\right) + W_2 - W_1}{\dfrac{W_3 - W_4}{G - 1} \times G} \times 100$

$w = \left[\left(\dfrac{W_2 - W_1}{W_3 - W_4}\right)\left(\dfrac{G - 1}{G}\right) - 1\right] \times 100$

W_1 = wt. of empty pycnometer

W_2 = wt. of pyc + soil

W_3 = wt. of pyc + water + soil

W_4 = wt. of pyc + water

Procedure :

1. Add some known quantity of water in oven dried soil whose weight is known. Mix the soil with water thoroughly.

2. Repeat the steps from 1 to 4 of part (a) of this experiment. Put the values of W_is and G in formula and find out the value of w.

3. Take some representative sample of soil. First weigh the empty container then put the sample in it and weigh it. The values are U_1, U_2 respectively.

4. Now put the container in an oven to dry the sample. After 24 hours weigh the container with dry soil in it. Mark it with U_3.

    The water content is

$$w = \frac{U_2 - U_3}{U_3 - U_1}$$

    Compare with the value obtained by pycnometer method.

5. For more than one water content values repeat the steps from 1 to 4 of this experiment and compare the values obtained by different methods for a value of w.

Observations :

For water content

		1	2	3
1.	Wt. of pyc. (W_1 gm)			
2.	Wt. of pyc + wet soil (W_2 gm)			
3.	Wt. of pyc + wet soil water (W_3 gm)			
4.	Wt. of pyc + water (W_4 gm)			

Container No.

	1	2	3
Wt. of container (U_1 gm)			
Wt. of container + wet soil sample (U_2 gm)			
Wt. of container + dry soil sample (U_3 gm)			

Result :

	1	2	3
Water content (i)			
(ii)			

Precautions :

1. Water must be as pure as possible. If available take distilled water only, because impurities in water may lead to wrong observations.
2. There should not be any air bubbles in soil (in pycnometer method) and after that up the pycnometer upto the hole of conical cap.

Limitations :

1. This pycnometer method is used in coarse grain soils only.

Questions :

1. If the temperature at the time of performing the experiment is different from room temperature (i.e., 27°C) how will you determine the specific gravity?
2. Can you use kerosene oil in place of water to determine the specific gravity? If yes, then in what case it must be used and what are the changes that must be made in formula?
3. What is the difference between the specific gravity of soil grains and soils?
4. What is the standard temperature at which the value of specific gravity is alive?

Check :

Typical values of *G* which can be used as a guide in determining whether test results are correct, are as follows :

Type of Soil	*G*
Sand	2.65-2.67
Silty sand	2.67-2.70
Inorganic clay	2.70-2.80
Soils, with Mices E iron	2.75-3.00
Organic soils	Variable best may be under 2.00

Experiment No. 3

Object :

Determination of Atterberg's Limits.

A. Determination of Liquid Limit

Apparatus/Equipment :

Mechanical liquid limit device (Cassangrande type) consisting of a brass cup and carriage mounted on base Micarta Number 221A; grooving tool 'a' (Cassangrande or B.S. tool) and grooving tool 'b' (ASTM tool); porcelain evaporating dish, about 12 cm in diameter or marble plate 30 cm square; flexible spatula, with blade about 8 cm long and 2 cm wide; balance; air tight containers to determine water content; thermostatically controlled oven to maintain temperature between 105° to 110°C; wash bottle containing distilled water; 425 micron sieve; desicator.

Theoretical background :

Liquid limit is the minimum water content at which the soil is still in liquid state but has a small shearing strength against flowing. In other words it is the water content at which soil suspension gains an infinitesimal strength from zero strength. In the standard liquid limit apparatus for practical purposes, it is the minimum water content at which part of soil cut by a groove of standard dimensions, will flow together for a distance of 12 mm (1/2 inch) under an impact of 25 blows.

Procedure :

1. By means of the gauge on the handle of the grooving tool and the adjustment plate, adjust the height through which the cup is lifted and dropped so that the point on the cup which comes in contact with the base falls through exactly 1 cm when the handle is rotated by one revolution. When the adjustment is complete, secure the adjustment plate by tightening its screws.

2. Take about 120 g of the specimen passing through the 425 micron sieve, and mix it thoroughly with distilled water in the evaporating dish or on the marble plate so that uniform paste is formed. Leave the soil for sufficient time so that water may permeate throughout the soil mass. In the case of fat clays, this measuring time may be upto 24 hours. For an average soil, thorough mixing for 15 to 30 minutes is sufficient. The amount of water to be added depends completely on the type of soil.

3. Take a portion of the paste with spatula and place it in the centre of the cup so that it is almost half filled. Level flat the top of the wet soil symmetrically with the spatula, so that it is parallel to the rubber base with a maximum depth of the soil being 1 cm.

4. With the help of grooving tool 'a', the paste in the cup is divided along the cup diameter (through the centre line of the can follower), by holding the tool normal to the surface of the cup and drawing it firmly across. Thus a V shaped groove 2 mm vide at the bottom and 11 mm at the top and 8 mm deep will be formed. However, in the case of sandy soil tool 'a' does not form a neat groove and hence tool 'b' is used.

5. Turn the handle of the apparatus at the rate of 2 revolutions per second, until the two parts of the soil

come in contact with the bottom of the groove along a distance of 10 mm. Record the no. of blows required to cause the groove close for approximate length of 10 mm.

6. Collect a representative slice of soil by moving the spatula widthwise from one edge to the other edge of the soil cake at right angles to the groove, including the portion of the groove in which the soil flowed together, and put it in an air tight container. Its water content is then determined.

7. Remove the remaining soil from the cup and mix it with the soil left earlier on the marble plate (or evaporating dish). Change the consistency of the mix by either adding more water or leaving the soil paste to dry as the case may be and repeat steps 3, 4, 5 and 6. Note the number of revolutions to close the groove and keep the soil for water content determination. These operations are repeated for 3 or 4 more additional trials. The soil paste in these operations should be of such consistency that the number of revolutions or drops to close the groove is 25 ± 10.

Observations :

	Determination No.		1	2	3	4
1.	Container No.					
2.	Wt. of container	(g)				
3.	No. of blows					
4.	Wt. of container + wet soil	(g)				
5.	Wt. of container + dry soil	(g)				
6.	Wt. of water	(g)				
7.	Wt. of oven dry soil	(g)				
	Water content = $\dfrac{(6)}{(7)}$	(%)				

Calculations :

Plot the flow curve on a semilog graph with water content as the ordinate and no. of blows as abscissa. The water content corresponding to 25 blows is taken as the liquid limit of the soil.

Results :

Liquid Limit, w_L (from graph) =

Flow index or slope of the curve, I_f (from graph) $= \dfrac{w_1 - w_2}{\log_{10} \dfrac{n_1}{n_2}}$

w_1 = water content corresponding to blows n_1

w_2 = water content corresponding to blows n_2

Precautions :

The test should always proceed from drier to the wetter condition of the soil.

B. Determination of Plastic Limit

Apparatus/Equipment :

All items of part A except first two items and a rod of 3 mm diameter.

Theoretical background :

Plastic limit is the minimum water content at which a soil just begins to crumble when rolled into a thread of 3 mm in diameter. This water content is in between the plastic and semi-solid states of soil.

Procedure :

1. Take about 20 g of air dried soil from a thoroughly mixed portion of the soil passing 425 micron IS sieve. Mix it on the marble plate with sufficient distilled water to make it plastic enough to be shaped into a ball. Leave the plastic soil mass for some time to mature. For some fat clays, the plastic soil mass may be left for 24 hours to allow water to permeate throughout the soil mass.
2. Take about 8 g of plastic soil, make a ball of it and roll it on the marble (or glass) plate with just sufficient pressure to roll the mass into the thread of uniform diameter throughout its length. When the diameter or thread has decreased to 3 mm the specimen is kneaded together and rolled out again. Continue this process until the thread just crumbles at 3 mm diameter.
3. Collect the crumbled soil thread in the airtight container and keep it for the water content determination. The test is repeated twice more. Thus, three readings are obtained for the determination.
4. Also, determine the natural water content of the soil sample obtained from the field.

Observations and Result :

Determination No.		1	2	3	4
Container No.					
Wt. of container	(g)				
Wt. of container + wet soil	(g)				
Wt. of container + oven dry soil	(g)				
Wt. of water	(g)				
Wt. of dry soil	(g)				
Water content = $\dfrac{\text{wt. of water}}{\text{wt. of dry soil}}$	(%)				

Plastic limit w_p =   Av. water content =

Calculations :

1. Plastic limit =
2. Plasticity index $I_p = w_L - w_p$
3. Flow index I_f (from Part A of Exp.) =
4. Toughness index $I_T = \dfrac{I_p}{I_f} =$

C. Determination of Shrinkage Limit

Apparatus/Equipment :

Evaporating dish, shrinkage dish, glass cup, glass plates, spatula, straight edge, 425 micron IS sieve, balances, oven, mercury, desicator, wash bottle.

Theoretical background :

Shrinkage limit is the water content at which further reduction in it will not lead to decrease in volume of soil mass.

Let,

Wt. of wet soil = W_1 gm

Vol. of wet soil V_1 = Vol. of dish

Wt. of dry soil = W_2 gm

Vol. of dry soil = V_2 gm

Loss of volume = $V_1 - V_2$

Wt. of water at shrinkage limit ? ...(i)

Loss of wt. of water till the start of shrinkage limit = $\rho_w (V_1 - V_2)$ ...(ii)

Total loss of water = $W_1 - W_2$ gm ...(iii)

Therefore,

Wt. of water at shrinkage limit = total loss of water – loss of water at the start of shrinkage limit

$$= W_1 - W_2 - \rho_r (V_1 - V_2)$$ ...(iv)

Shrinkage limit = water content at shrinkage $u = 100 \times \dfrac{W_1 - W_2 - \rho_w (V_1 - V_2)}{W_2}$

Shrinkage limit $= \dfrac{W_1 - W_2}{W_2} - \dfrac{\rho_w (V_1 - V_2)}{W_2} \times 100$

$\dfrac{W_1 - W_2}{W_2} = w = $ water content

$\rho_w = 1$

$W_2 = W_d$

$V_1 = V$

$V_2 = V_d$

Shrinkage limit $= w - \dfrac{V - V_d}{W_d} \times 100$

Procedure :

1. *Preparation of soil paste.* Take about 100 g of soil sample from a thoroughly mixed portion of the material passing 425 micron IS sieve.
2. Place about 30 g of the above sample in evaporating dish and mix it thoroughly with distilled water. Water added should be sufficient to fill the voids in the soil completely and make the soil wet enough to be readily worked into the shrinkage dish without entrapping air bubbles.
3. Clean the shrinkage dish and determine its weight accurate to 0.1 g. To determine its volume, place the shrinkage dish in the evaporating dish and fill it with mercury. Remove the excess mercury by pressing the glass plate firmly on its top taking care that no air is entrapped. Wipe off, carefully, the mercury which is adhering to the outside of the shrinkage dish. Carefully transfer the mercury of the

shrinkage dish to the other evaporating dish, and then determine the weight of mercury accurate to 0.1 g. The weight of mercury divided by its unit weight would give the volume of the shrinkage dish, which is also the volume of the wet soil.

4. *Filling the shrinkage dish with wet soil.* Coat the inside of the shrinkage dish with a thin layer of silicon grease or vaseline. Strike off the excess soil paste with a straight edge. Wipe off the soil adhering to the outside of the dish.

5. *Determination of wet and dry weight of soil.* Weigh immediately the shrinkage dish plus the wet soil, accurate to 0.1 g. Keep the shrinkage dish open to air until the colour of soil sample turns from dark to light. Keep the shrinkage dish in the oven and thus dry the soil sample at constant temperature at 105°C to 110°C. Cool the dish in a desicator and weigh immediately.

6. *Determination of volume of dry soil.* To determine the volume of dry soil, keep the glass cup in the evaporating dish. Fill the cup to over flowing with mercury. Remove the excess mercury by pressing the glass plate with the three prongs firmly over the top of the cup. Transfer the cup carefully to another evaporating dish, carefully wiping off any mercury which may be adhering to the outside of the cup. Place the oven dried soil pat on the surface of mercury in the cup and carefully force the pat into the mercury by pressing it by the same glass plate containing three prongs. Press the plate firmly on the top of the cup. Collect carefully the displaced mercury and weigh to an accuracy of 0.01 g. The volume of the dry soil is then determined by dividing this weight by the unit weight of mercury.

Observations :

	Determination No.		1	2	3
(a)	Water content of wet soil				
1.	Shrinkage dish No.				
2.	Wt. of shrinkage dish	(g)			
3.	Wt. of shrinkage dish + wet soil	(g)			
4.	Wt. of shrinkage dish + dry soil	(g)			
5.	Wt. of dry soil (W_d)	(g)			
6.	Wt. of water	(g)			
7.	Water content of soil (w) (ratio) $= \dfrac{(6)}{(5)}$				
(b)	Volume of wet soil				
8.	Evaporating dish No.				
9.	Wt. of mercury filling shrinkage dish + wt. of evaporating dish	(g)			
10.	Wt. of evaporating dish	(g)			
11.	Wt. of mercury filling evaporating dish	(g)			
12.	Vol. of wet soil $V = \dfrac{(11)}{13.6}$	(cm^3)			
(c)	Volume of dry soil				
13.	Evaporating dish No.				
14.	Wt. of mercury displaced by dry soil + wt. of evaporating dish	(g)			
15.	Wt. of evaporating dish	(g)			
16.	Wt. of mercury displaced by dry soil	(g)			
17.	Vol. of dry soil $V_d = \dfrac{(16)}{13.6}$	(cm^3)			

Calculations :

Shrinkage Limit.

$$w_S = w - \frac{V - V_d}{W_d} \times 100 =$$

Results :

Shrinkage Limit (Remoulded Sample) =

Questions :

1. Why do you use mercury only to determine the volume of wet and dry soil pat? Can you use any other compound?
2. Is it possible to get the true value of plastic limit?
3. How the plastic limit is defined to determine it in the laboratory?
4. What is plastic state? What is the state of soil at plastic limit? Do different soils at their plastic limits have the same state?
5. What is the consistency of soil at plastic limit? Do different soils at their plastic limits have different consistencies?
6. Is plastic limit a natural or conventional soil index?
7. What is the degree of saturation at plastic limit?
8. What happens when water content of a soil is reduced from liquid limit to plastic limit?
9. Do different soils have the same shear strength at their plastic limits? Justify.
10. What are the practical applications of plastic limit, plasticity index and relative plasticity index of soils?
11. Why do you use the soil passing from 425 microns sieve to determine the plastic limit while its value is used to classify only the fine grained soils, which is passing from 75 microns sieve?
12. If a thread of 5 mm is made instead of 3 mm then what is the effect on plastic limit?
13. What is the degree of saturation at shrinkage limit?
14. Does volume increase on addition of water content at shrinkage limit?
15. What are the factors affecting the value of shrinkage limit?
16. If air bubble is left during filling the wet soil in the shrinkage dish, what is its effect on shrinkage limit?

Values (Standard) :

Unit weight of mercury = 13.53 g/cc
Unit weight of water = 1.00 g/cc

Experiment No. 4

Object :

To determine grain-size distribution of coarse grained soil by sieving.

Apparatus :

Balances, set of IS sieves, mechanical sieve-shaker.

Theoretical background :

The grain size of soil can be determined by the sieve plate aperture size used in the process of sieving. The weight of soil retained in each stack is used to get the percentage finer "by weight" and obtain the grain size distribution and hence the distribution.

Procedure :

For sandy to fine grained soils, the recommended sieve stack (in order from top to bottom) is as follows :
   4.75 mm
   2.00 mm
   1.00 mm
    600 microns
    425 microns
    300 microns
    212 microns
    150 microns
    75 microns
Remove the stack of sieves from the shaker and obtain the weight of material retained on each sieve.

Compute the per cent retained on each sieve by dividing the weight retained on each sieve by original sample weight w_S. Compute the per cent passing (or per cent finer) by starting with 100% and subtracting the per cent retained on each sieve as cumulative procedure. Make a semilogarithmic plot of grain size versus per cent finer.

Observations and Calculations :

Weight of dry soil sample W_s =

S. No.	IS Sieve	Particle size D (mm)	Weight retained (g)	% weight retained	Cumulative % retained	Cumulative % finer

Result :

From the graph get the following

(a) Coefficient of uniformity $C_u = \dfrac{D_{60}}{D_{10}} =$

(b) Coefficient of concavity curvature $C_c = \dfrac{(D_{30})^2}{(D_{10} \times D_{60})}$

(c) Classify the soil sample as per MIT and Indian Standards classification.

Note : D refers to the grain size, or apparent diameter, of the soil particles and the subscript of (10, 30, 60) denotes the percent that is smaller. For example, if D_{10} is equal to 0.15 mm, it will mean that 10% of sample grains are smaller than 0.15 mm.

Precautions :

1. Take the dry soil only. If it is wet, dry it in oven.
2. The time of shaking must be according to weight of soil sample taken.
3. After the shaking obtain the weight of material retained on each sieve. Sum these weights and detect any loss of soil. If the loss of weight is more than 2% of initial weight then repeat the whole experiment carefully.

Limitations :

1. It is only for coarse grained soil.
2. It does not provide information on the shape of the soil grains i.e. whether they are angular or rounded or flaky etc. It only yields information on grains that passes with proper orientation through openings of certain size.

Questions :

1. What does C_u indicate?
2. What is the significance of C_c?
3. Does MIT classification and IS classification give coherent results?

Experiment No. 5

Object :

To determine the grain size distribution by hydrometer.

Apparatus :

Hydrometer, thermometer, balance, etc.

Theoretical background :

This test is based on Stoke's law. According to this, terminal velocity is given by

$$v = \frac{\rho_s - \rho_w}{18\,u} D^2$$

ρ_s = unit wt. of solid particles

ρ_w = unit wt. of water

u = viscosity of water

D = diameter of solid particles

$$D = \sqrt{\frac{18\,uv}{\rho_s - \rho_w}}$$

If a particle of diameter D falls through a distance h in time t

$$v = h/t$$

$$D = \sqrt{\frac{18\,uh}{(\rho_s - \rho_w)\,t}}$$

The specific gravity of suspension is determined by hydrometer at a particular depth.

The height h can be written in terms of h_1, h_0, V_H, A_j

$$h = h_1 + h_0 + \frac{V_H}{2\,A_j} - \frac{V_H}{A_j}$$

where $\dfrac{V_H}{2\,A_j}$ = rise in the level of water at the centre of bulb of hydrometer. Since below the centre of bulb of hydrometer the rise in the level is due to half of the volume of hydrometer only.

$\dfrac{V_H}{A_j}$ = total rise or rise in the surface of suspension. Here full volume (inserted part only) of hydrometer is taken into account. The reading of hydrometer gives the sp. gravity of the suspension

$$= \frac{\text{wt. of water/cc} + \text{immersed wt. of solid/cc}}{\text{wt. of water/cc}}$$

$$= 1 + \text{immersed wt. of solid/cc}$$

from the reading of hydrometer the sp. gravity is determined as given below.

Let R is the reading (corrected) of hydrometer. Specific gravity $= 1 + \dfrac{R}{1000}$

$$\therefore \quad 1+\frac{R}{1000} = 1 + \text{immersed wt. of solid/cc}$$

Immersed wt. of solid/cc. $= W_d\left(\dfrac{G-1}{G}\right)$

Therefore

$$W_d = \frac{R}{1000}\left(\frac{G}{G-1}\right)$$

G = specific gravity of solid

W_d = wt. of solids/cc at depth h after time t.

Hence percentage of particles smaller than D is equal to

$$\frac{W_d}{\text{wt. of solid/cc in original suspension}} \times 100$$

Procedure :

Calibration of hydrometer

1. Immerse the hydrometer in jar full of water and note down the rise in level of water. Increased volume of water corresponds to temperature of hydrometer.
2. Measure the distance between any two graduation marks on jar and find the volume included in between these two graduation. Ratio of this volume and height gives the cross sectional area A of jar.
3. Calculate the effective height for each major calibration mark and draw the calibration curve between effective height and hydrometer reading.
4. Weigh about 50 gm to 100 gm of soil and pour it in jar filled with water. Then mix some dispersing agent in suspension in jar to assure uniform density of suspension.
5. Place a suitable cover on the top of jar and shake it vigorously end over end. Stop shaking and allow it to settle. Remove the top cover and start stop watch immediately.
6. Insert the hydrometer and take reading after periods of 1/2, 1, 2, 4 minutes. Take out hydrometer and rinse it with distilled water.
7. Reinsert the hydrometer and take the reading for 8, 15, 30 minutes, 1 hr, 2 hr, 4 hr. After each reading hydrometer should be rinsed.

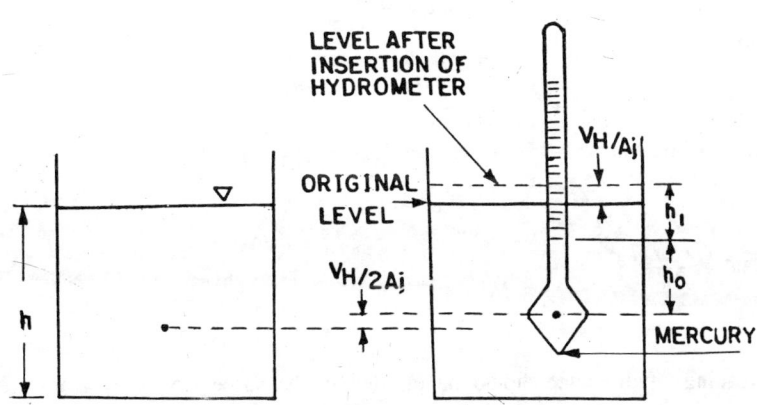

Observations :

$A =$ $G =$

$V_H =$ $h_0 =$

Time	Hydrometer Reading	h_1	h

Calculation Table :

Time	R	h	W_d	% finer	Particle size D

h_1 should be determined by calibration curve from calculation table. Draw the graph between particle size and percentage finer.

Determine from graph,

$D_{60} =$

$D_{10} =$

and find out uniformity coefficient.

Result :

Uniformity constant $= \dfrac{D_{60}}{D_{10}} =$

Precautions :

After first four readings hydrometer should be inserted in the suspension only a few second before the reading is to be taken.

Limitation :

It is for fine soil only.

Questions :

1. What does uniformity coefficient indicate?
2. What type of corrections can be done in hydrometer reading?
3. What is the effect of using erroneous value of G being 2.60 when the correct value is 2.70?
4. What is hydrometer and sedimentation analysis?
5. What is Stoke's law and what are its assumptions?
6. How does Stoke's law help in hydrometer analysis?
7. What is the effect of the size of the soil particles on their velocities in soil water suspension?
8. State two or more uses of hydrometer test data.
9. What is the role of dispersing/deflocculating agent in hydrometer analysis? Name the most common used in hydrometer analysis. How is its solution prepared?

Experiment No. 6

Object :

Determination of compaction properties of a sample of soil.

Apparatus :

Metal rammer, steel straight edge, 20 mm and 4.75 mm IS sieves, balance, Water content containers, mixing equipment, measuring cylinder of glass, Proctor's needle.

Theoretical background :

Compaction is the process in which soil particles are rearranged in a closer state by impact loading and air is expelled from voids. The dry density of soil changes with its water content. Initially density increase with increase in water content since this moisture helps in bringing the soil particles closer. If we go on adding the water then after a certain stage dry density of soil starts decreasing, since the excess of water starts occupying the space that could have been occupied by soil grains under compaction. Thus the water content at which the dry density of soil is maximum is called optimum water content.

$$\rho_d = \frac{\rho_s}{1+w}$$

ρ_d = dry density

ρ_s = bulk density

w = water content

$$\rho_s = \frac{\text{total weight}}{\text{total volume}} = \frac{\text{wt. of water} + \text{wt. of soil}}{\text{vol. of solid} + \text{vol. of voids}} = \frac{W_w + W_s}{V_v + V_s} = \frac{W_s\left(1 + \dfrac{W_w}{W_s}\right)}{V_s\left(1 + \dfrac{V_v}{V_s}\right)}$$

$$\rho_s = \frac{W_s(1+w)}{V_s(1+e)}$$

e = void ratio = $\dfrac{V_v}{V_s}$

w = water content = $\dfrac{W_s}{V_s}$

Sp. gravity $G = \dfrac{W_s}{V_s}$

$$\rho_s = \frac{G(1+w)}{(1+e)} \qquad \text{or,} \qquad \frac{\rho_s}{1+w} = \rho_d = \frac{G}{1+e}$$

$$\therefore \quad e = \frac{G}{\rho_d} - 1$$

Procedure :

1. Take a representative sample weighing approximately 20 kg of thoroughly mixed dried soil passing 4.75 mm (or 20 mm) IS sieve. Add enough water to bring its water content upto 7% (sandy soil) or 10% (clayey soils) less than the estimated optimum moisture content.

2. Clean the mould and fix it to the base. Take the empty weight of mould and base nearest to 1 g.

3. Attach the collar to the mould. The inside of the mould should be grease.

4. Mix the matured soil thoroughly. Take out about 2½ kg of the soil and compact it in the mould in three equal layer, each layer being given 25 blows from the rammer weighing 2.6 kg, dropping from a height of 310 mm if 1000 ml mould is used. If, however the 2250 ml mould is used about 5 kg of soil should be taken, and should be compacted in three equal layers, each layer being given 56 blows from the rammer weighing 2.6 kg dropping from a height of 310 mm. The blows should be uniformly distributed over the surface of each layer. Each layer of the compacted soil should be scored with a spatula before putting the soil for the succeeding layer. The amount of soil used should be just sufficient to fill the mould leaving about 5 mm to be struck off when the collar is removed. Find the penetration resistance of compacted soil, using the Proctor's needle.

5. Remove the collar and cut the excess soil with the help of straight edge. Clean the mould from outside and weigh it to the nearest gram. Take out the soil from the mould. Cut it in the middle and keep a representative soil specimen for water content determination.

6. Repeat steps 4 and 5 for about five or six times, using a fresh part of the soil specimen and after adding a higher water content than the preceding specimen.

Observations :

Determination No.		1	2	3	4	5	6	7
(a) Density								
Wt. of mould + compacted soil	(g)							
Wt. of mould	(g)							
Wt. of compacted soil	(g)							
Bulk density								
(b) Water content								
Wt. of container + wet soil	(g)							
Wt. of container + dry soil	(g)							
Wt. of water	(g)							
Wt. of container	(g)							
Wt. of dry soil	(g)							
Water content	(%)							
Dry Density =								

Calculations :

1. The dry density of the compacted soil is calculated as follows :

$$\rho_d = \frac{\rho_s}{1+w}$$

   A curve showing the relationship between dry density and water content is to be plotted. The water content corresponding to maximum dry density is to be found from the curve.

2. The void ratio is found from the relation

$$e = \frac{G}{\rho_d} - 1$$

   where G = specific gravity and ρ_d = dry density of soil.

3. On the same plot, a curve is drawn between penetration resistance and water content.

Result :

   The optimum water content is _____

   Max. dry density _____

Questions :

1. On what factors does optimum moisture content depend for a given soil? Explain.
2. Prove that ratio of compactive energy imparted in modified test to that of standard test is 4.55 : 1, when both the tests have same mould.

Experiment No. 7

Object :

To determine the permeability of soil.

Apparatus :

Jodhpur permeameter, mixing pan, balance, stop watch, container for water content determination.

Theoretical background :

The property of material which permits fluids to percolate through its voids is called permeability. According to Darcy's law, in the laminar range the velocity of percolation is proportional to the hydraulic gradient.

$V \propto i$

$V = K i$

$AV = K A i$

$AV =$ flow rate $= Q = K A i$

$K = \dfrac{Q L}{h A}$

$i =$ hydraulic gradient $= \dfrac{h}{L}$

$A =$ cross-sectional area of soil mass perpendicular to the direction of flow

$V =$ velocity of flow

$h =$ head loss in a distance L along the flow path

If the head is not constant and the rate of fall is $\dfrac{dh}{dt}$ then

$$\text{flow rate } Q = -a \frac{dh}{dt}$$

$$-a \frac{dh}{dt} = K \frac{h}{L} A$$

$$\int_{h_1}^{h_2} -\frac{a}{h} dh = \int_0^t \frac{KA}{L} dt$$

$$a \ln \frac{h_1}{h_2} = \frac{KAt}{L}$$

$$K = \frac{al}{At} \ln \frac{h_1}{h_2}$$

$a =$ cross sectional area of stand pipe

$t =$ time of flow

$h_1 =$ initial head

$h_2 =$ final head

Procedure :

A. Constant Head Method

(a) Preparation of specimen :

1. Take about 800 to 1000 gm of soil and mix with water so that its water content rises to optimum water content.
2. Grease the mould. Assemble the dynamic permeameter. Place the mould upside down on the dynamic compaction base and weigh the assembly. Put 3 cm collar to the other end.
3. Compact the wet soil in two layers by applying 15 blows to each layer with 2.5 kg ramming rod. Remove the collar and trim off the excess soil and weigh the assembly filled with soil and determine the weight of the soil.
4. Place the filter paper or fine wire mesh on the top of specimen and fix the perforated base plate on it.
5. Turn the specimen upside down. Remove the compaction plate and place the perforated plated on the top of the specimen and fix up the sealing and top cap.

(b) Saturation of compacted specimen :

Place the permeameter mould in the vacuum desicator and open air release valve. Fill the desicator with desired water such that it reaches well above the top cap. Apply the vacuum and increase it gradually to about 70 cm of mercury.

Testing :

1. Place the mould in bottom tank and fill it with water upto its outlet.
2. Connect the outlet of constant head tank to the inlet of permeameter. Adjust the head by either adjusting the relative height of mould and constant head tank or by raising or lowering the air in-take tube within the head tank.
3. Run the test for some convenient time interval.

   Note the duration of test by stop watch. Collect the water (V cc) in a beaker flowing from outlet of bottom tank and measure it.

Observations :

$h =$

$L =$

$A =$

$t =$

V I   test $=$

      II   test $=$ } $V_{av} =$

      III   test $=$

$K =$

Test temperature $=$

Permeability at 27°C $=$

Calculations :

$$Q = \frac{V}{t}$$

$$K = \frac{V}{t} \times \frac{1}{h} \times \frac{1}{A}$$

Result :

   $K =$

B. Falling Head Method

Preparation and saturation of specimen are same as that of constant head method.

Testing :

   1. Keep the permeameter mould assembly in the bottom tank and fill it upto its outlet.
   2. Connect inlet of mould to the stand pipe filled with water. Permit water to flow for some time until steady state of flow is reached.
   3. Note the time required for water level in the stand pipe to fall from some initial value to some final value.
   4. Repeat the step 3 for two or three times for same initial and final head value.

Determination of *a* :   Collect water contained in between two graduations (of the stand pipe) of known distance apart, weigh it and determine the inside area of stand pipe.

Observations :

   a = area of stand pipe =
   A = area of soil specimen =
   h_1 = initial head in stand pipe =
   h_2 = final head in stand pipe
   t_1 =
   t_2 =
   t_3 =
   Average t =

Calculations :

$$K = \frac{al}{At} \ln \frac{h_1}{h_2}$$

Result :

   $K =$

Precautions : Increase the cacousion slowly and in every increment sufficient time should be given to escape the air bubbles off the specimen without vibrating the specimen.

Limitations :   Generally this apparatus is used for fine grained (pervious) soil only.

Questions :

   1. How does the pore effect the permeability?
   2. Does cohesion of soil play any role in the determination of permeability?
   3. Compare the values of permeability K obtained from both methods and state the probable cause for any difference in the two values.
   4. Does temperature play any significant role in computing the permeability?

Experiment No. 8

Object :

Determination of consolidation properties of soil.

Apparatus :

Fixed ring type consolidometer, suitable loading device for applying vertical loading, dial gauge, balance, thermostatically controlled oven, containers, mixing basin, glass plate, filter paper, stop watch.

Theoretical background :

The process of compression resulting from long term steady load and gradual reductions of pore space by escaping of pore water is termed as consolidation. The permeability of an undisturbed sample of clay is determined directly at several different void ratios while running a consolidation test.

Procedure :

(a) Preparation of soil specimen :

1. *Preparation of specimen from undisturbed soil samples.* The undisturbed sample from the field may be circular (at least 1 cm in diameter) or a block sample. Clean the specimen ring and weigh it empty. Cut off about 3 to 5 cm of soil specimen from one end of the sample by pressing with hands and carefully removing the material around the ring. The soil specimen so obtained should project about 1 cm from either side of the ring. Trim the sample smooth and flush at the top and bottom of the ring by using glass plates. Clean the ring from outside and weigh. Keep three specimens from the soil trimmings for water content determination.

2. *Preparation of specimen from representative soil samples.* If the consolidation properties are to be determined from a disturbed soil sample, soil is compacted at the desired water content and density, in a separate large mould, and then the specimen is cut as explained in step (1) above.

(b) Preparation of mould assembly and sample :

1. Saturate the porous stones either by boiling in distilled water for about 15 minutes or by keeping them submerged in distilled water for 4 to 8 hours. Wipe away excess water. Moisture all surfaces of the consolidometer which are to be enclosed.

2. Assemble the consolidometer with the soil specimen (in the ring) and porous stones at top and bottom of the specimen providing a filter paper between soil specimen and porous stone. Position the pressure pad centrally on the top porous stone.

3. Mount the mould assembly on the loading frame and centre it such that the applied load is axial.

4. Position the dial gauge to measure vertical compression of the specimen. The dial gauge holder should be so set that the dial is near the beginning of its release run, allowing sufficient margin for the swelling of the soil, if any.

5. Connect the mould assembly to the water reservoir and allow the sample to be saturated. The level of water in the reservoir is at about the same level as the specimen.

6. Apply an initial setting load to the assembly. The magnitude of this load should be chosen by trail

such that there is no swelling. It should not be less than 50 gm/cm^2 for ordinary soil (or 25 g/cm^2 for very soft soils). The load should be allowed to stand until there is no change in dial gauge reading for two consecutive hours or for a maximum of 24 hours.

(c) Consolidation test :

1. Note the final dial reading under the initial setting load. Apply first load of intensity of 5.1 kg/cm^2 and start the stop watch simultaneously with loading. Record the dial gauge readings at various time intervals indicated in the observation table. The dial gauge readings are taken until 90% consolidation in reached. Primary consolidation is generally reached within 24 hours.

2. At the end of the period, specified above, take the dial reading and time reading. Double the intensity and take dial readings at various time intervals. Repeat this procedure for successive load increments. The usual load intensities are as follows : 0.1, 0.2, 0.5, 1, 2, 4 and 8 kg/cm^2.

3. After the last loading is completed, reduce the load to 1/4 of the value of the last and allow it to stand for 24 hours. Reduce the load further in steps of 1/4th of the previous intensity till an intensity of 0.1 kg/cm^2 is reached. Take the final reading of the dial gauge.

4. Reduce the load to the initial setting load, keep it for 24 hours and note the final dial readings.

5. Quickly dismantle the specimen assembly and remove the excess surface water on the soil specimen by blotting and weigh the ring with consolidation specimen. Dry the soil specimen in oven and determine its dry weight.

Observations and Result :

(a) For Pressure, Compression and Time

Empty weight of ring :

Dia. of ring :

Ht. of ring :

Area of O ring :

Volume of ring :

Sp. gravity of soil sample G :

Pressure Intensity (kg/cm^2)		0.1	0.2	0.5	1	2	4
Elapsed Time (min.)	$\sqrt{t}$	Dial Gauge Readings					
0	0						
0.25	0.5						
1	1						
2.25	1.5						
4	2						
6.25	2.25						
9	3						

Pressure Intensity (kg/cm^2)		0.1	0.2	0.5	1	2	4
Elapsed Time (min.)	$\sqrt{t}$	Dial Gauge Readings					
12.25	3.5						
16	4						
20.25	4.5						
25	5						
36	6						
49	7						
64	8						
81	9						
100	10						
121	11						
144	12						
169	13						
196	14						
225	15						
256	16						
289	17						
324	18						
361	19						
430	20						
500	22.4						
600	24.5						
1440	38						

(b) For Pressure Void Ratio

Applied pressure (kg/cm^2)	Final dial reading	Dial change H	Speci-men height $H_1 = H$	Drainage path $d = \frac{1}{4}(H_1 + H)$	Ht. of voids $H - H_s$	Voids ratio $e = \dfrac{H - H_s}{H_s}$	Fitting time		C_v (cm^2/min.)		Av. C_c	Remarks
							t_{50}	t_{90}	$\dfrac{0.197\, d^2}{t_{50}}$	$\dfrac{0.848\, d^2}{t_{90}}$		
0.1												
0.2												
0.5												
1.0												
2.0												
4.0												
8.0												
0												

(c) For Water Content

			Before Test	After Test
1.	Wt. of ring + wet soil	(g)		
2.	Wt. of ring + dry soil	(g)		
3.	Wt. of ring	(g)		
4.	Wt. dry soil (W_d)	(g)		
5.	Wt. of water	(g)		
6.	Water content 'w'			
7.	Degree of saturation $\dfrac{wG}{e}$			
8	Ht. of solids $H_s = \dfrac{W_d}{GA}$			

Calculations :

1. Height of solids (H_s) can be calculated as $H_s = \dfrac{W_d}{GA}$

2. Voids ratio $e = \dfrac{H - H_s}{H_s}$

3. Coefficient of consolidation

$$C_v = \frac{0.197\, d^2}{t_{50}} \quad \text{(log fitting method)}$$

$$C_v = \frac{0.848\, d^2}{t_{90}} \quad \text{(square root fitting method)}$$

In the log fitting method, a plot is made between dial reading and logarithm of time and the time corresponding to 50% consolidation is determined. In the square root fitting method, a plot is made between dial reading and the square root of time and the time corresponding to 90% consolidation is determined.

4. Compression index. A plot of void ratio e versus log 1 is made. The initial compression curve would be found to be a straight line and the slope of this line would give you the compression index G.

5. Coefficient of compressibility (av) $= \dfrac{0.435\, C_c}{\sigma_1}$

where σ_1 = average pressure for the increment.

6. Coefficient of permeability (k)

$$k = \frac{C_v\,(\text{av})\,\gamma_w}{1 + e}$$

Result :

Coefficient of consolidation

C_v (log fitting method) =

C_v (square root fitting method) =

Coefficient of compressibility a =

Coefficient of permeability k =

height of voids = $H - H_s$.

Questions :

1. What do you understand by coefficient of consolidation?
2. What do you mean by corrected zero point and its significance?
3. Why the consolidation test is required?

Experiment No. 9

Object :

To determine the California Bearing Ratio (CBR) of a compacted soil in unsoaked state.

Apparatus :

Mould, spacer disc, collar, rammer, compacting weight, annular slotted weight and other miscellaneous apparatus.

Theory :

CBR is the ratio of test load to the standard load expressed as percentage for a given penetration of the plunger.

$$CBR = \frac{\text{test load}}{\text{standard load}} \times 100$$

Test load is the penetration resistance at a particular penetration and standard load is the penetration resistance of the plunger into the standard sample (crushed stones) for that particular penetration.

Procedure :

Take about 4.5 to 5.5 kg soil, mix it with water to attain optimum moisture content. Fix the base plate to bottom of the mould and extension collar to its top. Insert the spacer disc over the base. Put the filter paper on the top of the displacer disc. Now compact the mixed soil in the mould either by light compaction or heavy compaction as explained in compaction test. Remove the collar and trim off the excess soil. Turn the mould upside down and remove base plate and displacer disc. Weigh the mould with compacted soil and find out the weight of soil and dry density of soil. Put the filter paper on the top of the compacted soil and clamp the perforated base plate on it.

Testing :

1. Place the surcharge weight on top of the soil specimen and place the mould assembly on the loading machine or compaction machine.

2. Put the penetration piston at the centre of the specimen with smallest possible load but in no case excess of 4 kg.

3. Set the stress and strain dial gauge to zero. Apply the load so that penetration ratio is approximately 1 to 5 mm/min. Note the load readings at various penetration, e.g., 0, 0.5, 1.0, 1.5, 2.0, 2.5, 3.0, 4.0, 5.0, 7.5, 10, 12.5 mm. Record maximum load and penetration before 12.5 mm penetration.

4. Take some soil from specimen for water content determination at the end of loading. This soil must be taken from the top 3 cm layer of the specimen.

Observations :

Surcharge wt. used =

Water content after penetration test =

Penetration Dial Readings (Penetration) (mm)	Load Dial Readings (Load) (kg)	Correct Load
0		
0.5		
1.0		
1.5		
2.0		
2.5		
3.0		
4.0		
5.0		
7.5		

Calculations :

Plot the graph for load versus penetration. If the curve is concave upward in starting then draw a tangent at the highest point and whereever it touches abscissa that will be corrected zero. With respect to this zero, mark the penetration value and find the correct load corresponding to them. Now the CBR —

$$CBR = \frac{\text{correct test load}}{\text{standard load}} \times 100$$

Standard Load :

Penetration	Load (1b)
0.1	3000
0.2	4500
0.3	5700
0.4	6900
0.5	7800

The CBR values are usually calculated for penetration of 2.5 mm and 5 mm. If CBR for 5 mm exceeds that for 2.5 mm, repeat the test. If identical results follow, CBR corresponding to 5 mm penetration should be taken for design.

If CBR value for 2.5 mm penetration is greater than that of 5 mm, 2.5 mm penetration CBR values is taken for design.

Result :

CBR Value =

At penetration =

Limitation :

This method is applicable to flexible pavements only.

Questions :

1. What is the function of surcharge load?
2. What do you mean by a flexible pavement?
3. What is the use of CBR value in design of pavement?
4. While in designing the pavement, if you come across the situation where water table is just below the subsoil and the subsoil is always saturated and submerged in water then what measure will you take in design to get the right value of CBR?

Experiment No. 10

Object :

To determine the shear parameters of cohesive soil by triaxial compression (undrained-unconsolidated) without measuring pore pressure.

Apparatus :

Triaxial cell, apparatus for applying and maintaining the desired fluid pressure in the cell, compression machine for application of deviator stress, dial gauge, split mould, rubber membrane stretcher, balance, stop watch, trimmer, etc.

Theoretical background :

A cylindrical soil specimen is subjected to direct stresses acting in three mutually perpendicular directions. Major principal stress acts in vertical direction and other two principal stresses namely intermediate and minor, act in horizontal directions. Minor principal stress is constant throughout the test and major principal circle is drawn for the stresses at failure. By Mohr circle shear strength of soil is determined.

Procedure :

Sample Preparation :
1. Mix the soil with water at desired water (optimum) content. Compact the soil properly in the split mould which should be oiled properly. Trim the excess soil and take out the specimen from mould carefully.
2. Determine the water content of this soil.
3. Then place the specimen on one of the end caps and put the other end cap on the top of the specimen.
4. Place the rubber membrane all round the specimen with the help of membrane stretcher.
5. Seal the rubber membrane with caps by means of rubber rings.

Compression Test :
1. Place the specimen on the pedestal in the triaxial cell.
2. Assemble the cell with the loading ram.
3. Admit the operating fluid in the cell and raise its pressure to the desired value. Adjust the loading machine to bring the loading ram a short distance away from the seat on the top cap of the specimen. Read the initial reading of load measuring dial gauge. Bring the loading ram just in contact with the seat on the top of specimen. Read the initial reading of dial gauge measuring axial compression.
4. Repeat the test on three or four specimens of same water content and same soil but under different cell pressure.

Specimen measurements :

Initial weight =   Final weight =

Initial water content =   Final water content =

Diameter =   Area =   Volume =

Speci-men	Comp. dial reading	Load gauge reading	Comp. of sample	Strain	Connected area	Load	Deviator stress $(\sigma_1 - \sigma_3)$	Vertical stress	Stress ratio
1.									
2.									
3.									

Sample	σ_3	$\sigma_1 - \sigma_3$	σ_1	σ_1/σ_3
1.				
2.				
3.				

σ_3 = cell pressure at failure

σ_1 = vertical stress at failure

$\sigma_1 - \sigma_3$ = deviator stress at failure

Calculations :

1. Plot $(\sigma_1 - \sigma_3)$ versus strain (ε) for each specimen.
2. Obtain the shear strength from Mohr circle and find out coefficient of cohesion also.

Result :

i)   Shear strength =

ii) Cohesion =

Questions :

1. What is meant by "area correction" of specimen? Apply this correction in your experiment.
2. What changes in the experiment are to be incorporated if pore pressure is also taken into consideration?

Experiment No. 11

Object :

To determine unconfined compressive strength of a soil specimen.

Apparatus :

Compression device, sample ejector, dial gauge, stop watch, oven, balance, etc.

Theoretical background :

The test is performed on cylindrical sample. Sample is subjected to direct compression until it fails.

Let the initial length = L_0

Change in length = ΔL

$\therefore$ axial strain = $\dfrac{\Delta L}{L_0}$

Initial area = A_0

Assuming volume of sample is constant throughout the test and area at failure is A_1

$\therefore$ $A_0 L_0 = A_1 L_1$

where $L_1 = L_0 - \Delta L$

Since compressive force is applied

$A_0 L_0 = A_1 (L_0 - \Delta L)$

$$A_1 = \frac{A_0 L_0}{L_0 - \Delta L} = \frac{A_0}{1 - \dfrac{\Delta L}{L_0}}$$

$\dfrac{\Delta L}{L_0}$ = strain

$$\text{Compressive stress} = \frac{\text{Load}}{\text{Area}}$$

$$= \frac{\text{Spring constant} \times \text{Spring expansion or contraction}}{\text{Area}}$$

$$\text{Compressive stress} = \frac{K}{A_0} \Delta L \left(1 - \frac{\Delta L}{L_0} \right)$$

Procedure :

1. Soil which is to be tested is mixed with water. This sample is then filled in the mould which is oiled in advance. The mould is having the same internal diameter as that of specimen which is to be tested. The mould is opened carefully and sample is taken out. Prepare two or three such samples for testing.
2. Measure the initial length and diameter of the specimen.
3. Put the specimen on bottom plate of the loading device. Adjust the upper plate to make contact with the specimen. Set the dial gauge (compression) at zero.

4. Compress the specimen until cracks are developed or the stress strain curve is well past its peak or until a vertical deformation of 20% is reached. Take the dial reading approximately at every 1 mm deformation of the specimen.

5. Repeat the steps from 2 to 5 for other soil sample.

6. Determine water content of each sample.

Observations :

1. Internal diameter of specimen (D_0) =
2. Initial length (L_0) =
3. Initial area (A_0) =
4. Initial density =
5. Initial water content =
6. Spring constant =

S. No.	Sample No.	Load in kg	Deformation in mm	Strain E %	Area A cm^2	Stress kg/cm^2

Calculations :

A plot is made between stress and strain for each soil sample. The maximum stress from curve gives the value of the unconfined compressive strength which is taken as the stress at 20% axial strain. Try to find the effect of water content on the compressive strength.

Result :

The unconfined compressive strength =

Limitation :

It is possible for cohesive soil only.

Questions :

1. Why is this test possible for cohesive soil only?
2. Why is it called quick test?

Experiment No. 12

Object :

To determine the shear strength of a cohesionless soil with the help of shear box test.

Apparatus :

1. Shear box equipment consisting of (a) shear box 60 mm^2 and 50 mm deep, divided into two parts horizontally with suitable spacing screws (b) container for shear box (c) grid plates, one plane and other perforated.
2. Loading frame.
3. Providing ring with dial gauge to measure shear force.
4. Dial gauge to measure horizontal displacement.

Theory :

Shear strength of soil is the ability to resist sliding along internal surfaces within a mass. The direct shear test is conducted on a soil in the idealized condition, i.e., the failure plane is forced to occur at a predetermined location. On this plane there are two stresses acting — a normal stress due to applied vertical load P_v and a shearing stress due to applied horizontal load P_h.

Thus $\sigma_n = \dfrac{P_v}{A}$ and $\tau = \dfrac{P_h}{A}$

where A is the nominal area of specimen (or of shear box)

$\tau = c + \sigma_n \tan \phi$ (c is zero for cohesionless soils)

As there are two unknown quantities, two values, as a minimum, of normal (applied) stress σ_n and shear (measured) stress τ will be required for solution.

Procedure :

1. Carefully assemble the shear box, keeping the grid plate at the bottom. The serrations of the grid plate should be placed at right angle to the direction of shear.
2. Place the soil sample in the shear box to about 5 mm from the top and place the grid plate and loading block on top of the soil.
3. Mount the shear box assembly on the load frame. Set the lower part of the shear box to bear against the load jack and upper part of the box to bear against proving ring. Set the dial of proving ring to zero. Attach the dial gauge to measure the shear displacement.
4. Put the loading yoke on top of loading block. Put normal weight on the hanger of loading yoke. Remove the shear box pins.
5. Start the horizontal (shear) loading and take the readings of load dial (of proving ring) and shear displacement dial. The rate of strain may vary from 1 to 2.5 mm per minute. Conduct the test till failure of sample.
6. Repeat the test for vertical loads of 5 kg, 7.5 kg, 15 kg, 30 kg and 40 kg.

Observations:

Area of soil specimen = (6×6) cm^2

Proving ring constant : 1 Div. = 0.6583×10^{-2} kg/cm^2

Displacement dial reading	Proving ring reading				
	5 kg	7.5 kg	15 kg	30 kg	40 kg
20					
40					
60					
80					
100					
120					
140					
160					
180					
200					
220					
240					
260					
280					
300					
320					
340					
360					
380					
400					

Calculations :

Test No.	Normal stress = $\dfrac{\text{Vertical load}}{36}$ (kg/cm^2)	Shear stress at failure = $0.6583 \times 10^{-2} \times$ proving ring dial reading at failure (kg/cm^2)	Shear displacement at failure
1.			
2.			
3.			
4.			

1. Plot the values of shear stress ε versus normal stress σ_n for the test. Construct a best fit straight line through the plotted points. Be sure to use same scale for both the ordinate (ε) and the abscissa (σ_n). Obtain the cohesion (if any) as the intercept with the ordinate axis and measure the slope of the line to obtain ϕ.

2. Plot ϕ versus shear displacement and find out the peak strength.

Results :

Cohesion 'e' =

Angle of internal friction 'ϕ' =

Precaution :

Rate of application of shear force must be constant in whole experiment.

Limitation:

The plane of failure is predetermined which may not be the weakest point.

Questions:

1. What are the factors which govern the angle of internal friction?

2. What is the critical void ratio?

Experiment No. 13

Object :

To determine cone bearing value.

Apparatus :

Proctor mould, a cone bearing value apparatus and loads.

Theory :

In this method a cone is allowed to fall on the soil which is placed in container. The penetration is correlated with shearing strength of soil. The resistance offered to penetration is correlated with shearing strength of the soil.

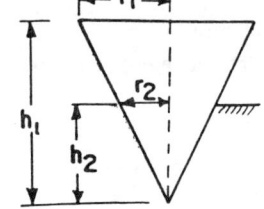

$$\text{Cone bearing value} = \frac{\text{Load}}{\text{Cross-section area of penetration at soil surface}}$$

$$= \frac{\text{self weight} + \text{Applied load}}{\pi \left(\dfrac{(r_1 h_2)^2}{h_1{}^2} \right)}$$

$$\frac{r_1}{r_2} = \frac{h_1}{h_2}$$

r_1, r_2, h_1, h_2 are as shown in figure.

Procedure :

Take 2.5 kg of the soil sample and add 12% of water in it. After mixing it thoroughly, it is put in the proctor's mould and filled in 3 layers compacting every layer 25 times. Then apex of cone bearing apparatus is kept in touch with the surface of the soil sample and the initial reading is taken. Load of 5 kg is put and final reading is noted. The operation is repeated with 10 kg, 20 kg and 40 kg loads.

Observations :

Initial Reading =   Self wt. =

S. No.	Load applied	Total load = Self wt. of cone + Applied load	Final reading	h_2 cm^2	Cone bearing value r_2
1.					
2.					
3.					

Calculations :

Av. cone bearing value $= \dfrac{\text{cone bearing value}}{3}$

Result :

Cone bearing value =

Limitation :

This test is recommended for cohesive soil only.

Question :

1. What happens if the cone is allowed to fall from a height of 30 cm having a load of 5 kg (total load)? What error will you encounter in such a situation?

Reference for Soil Mechanics Laboratory

1. ASTM (1960), Papers on Soils : Symposium on Atterberg Limits, Special Technical Publication (STP) No. 254, pp. 159-22⸠

2. Cassangrande, A. (1932), Research on the Atterberg Limits of Soils, Vol. 13, No. 8, October, pp. 121-136.

3. Fang H.Y. (1960), Rapid Determination of Liquid Limits of Soils by Flow Index Method, Bulletin No. 254, pp. 30-35.

4. Procter R.R. (1966), Fundamental Principles of Soil Compaction, Engineering News Record, Aug. 31, Sept. 7, pp. 21 and 28.

5. Johnson A.W. and Sallberg J.R. (1962), Factors Influencing Compaction Results, Bulletin No. 319, pp. 148.

6. Mitchel J.K., Hooper D.R. and Companella R.G. (1965), Permeability of Compacted Clay, Soil Mechanics and Foundation Division, July 4, pp. 41-65.

7. Cassangrande A. (1936), The Determination of the Pre-consolidation Load and its Practical Significance, Proceedings of First International Conference on Soil Mechanics and Foundation Engineering, Harvard, Vol. 3, pp. 60-64.

8. Crawford C.B. (1964), Interpretation of Consolidation Test, Soil Mechanics and Foundation Division, Sept. 5, pp. 87-102.

9. ASTM (1949-59), Triaxial Testing of Soils and Bituminous Mixtures, Special Technical Publication No. 106.

10. ASTM (1964), Symposium on Laboratory Testing of Soils, STP No. 361.

11. Bowles J.E., Engineering Properties of Soils and their Measurement, McGraw Hill Publishing Co., New York, second edition, 1978.

12. Lambe T.W., Soil Testing for Engineers, Wiley Eastern Limited, 4th edition reprinted, 1976.

13. Punmia, Dr. B.C., Soil Mechanics and Foundation Engineering, Nemchand and Brothers, Roorkee, second edition, 1982.

14. Prakash S. and Singh Bharat, Soil Mechanics and Foundation Engineering, Nemchand and Brothers, Roorkee, fifth edition reprinted, 1985.

15. Singhal R.P., A Text Book on Soil Mechanics and Foundation Engineering, Standard Book Depot, New Delhi, second reprinted edition, 1982.

SECTION 2

SURVEYING LABORATORY

Surveying is the skill of determining the relative position of points or objects by measurements of angles or distances. Some surveying experiments are explained in this section and their importance is as follows :

Tranversing is done to plot the details of any building or other structure. Whenever there is a need of precise measurement the triangulation survey is performed. It is a system of interconnected triangles are measured precisely. Plane tabelling is the method of surveying in which the field observation and plotting are done simultaneously. It is used to make manuscripts maps in the field. Contouring is used to determine the relative position of the point horizontally as well as vertically. A contour is an imaginary line on the ground joining the points of equal elevations.

The elevation of points along the central line of a railway, highway, canal or sewer is found by profile levelling. These railways or highways cannot be straight everywhere and thus their direction has to be changed. These directions are changed by curves. To layout the curves the curve plotting is used. These curves are traced out either by theodolite method or by chain and tape method.

Some times the accuracy is not much important but the speed of work is important. In these cases we use minor instruments for quick observations. e.g. hand level is used to determine the elevation of the point and sextant is used to find out the angles between two points. The slope of the ground is determines by Ceylon Ghat tracer.

Experiment No. 1

Object :

To determine the difference in elevations of two given points.

Apparatus :

Tilting level or Dumpy level, levelling staff.

Definitions of Terms :

M.S.L. (Mean sea level)

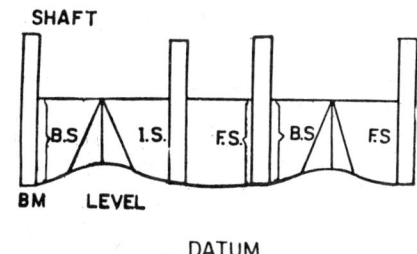

A Datum surface (line) : is any assumed surface or line from which the elevation of points are measured. M.S.L. is a convenient datum.

Elevation or reduced level : of a point is its vertical distance above or below the datum. It is known as reduced level (R.L.).

Value of R.L. is recorded :

(+) ve if above datum

(-) ve if below datum.

Bench mark (B.M.) : is a station or a point whose elevation is known.

Backsight (B.S.) : It is the first reading taken (after setting up the instrument) on a point of known elevation.

Foresight (F.S.) : It is the last reading taken, before shifting the instrument. It is usually on the point whose elevation is to be determined.

Intersight or intermediate sight (I.S.) : It is any other reading taken on a point of unknown elevation from the same set up of the level. All the readings taken between B.S. and F.S. are I.S.

Change point (C.P.) or Turning point (T.P.) : It is a point indicating the shifting of the level. At this point F.S. and B.S. both are taken.

Height of instrument (H.I.) : It is the elevation (or R.L.) of the plane of collimation when instrument is correctly levelled. It is also called "Height of plane of collimation".

Line of sight or line of collimation : It is the line passing through the optical centre of the objective, centre of cross wire passing the eye piece and entering the eye.

Procedure :

The procedure consists of :

    i) Making temporary adjustments with the level and taking the staff readings.

    ii) Working out the reduced levels of the points.

(a) The collimation system :

It consists in finding the elevation of the plane of collimation (H.I.) for every set-up of the instrument, and then obtaining the reduced levels of points with reference to the respective plane of collimation. To begin with, the elevation of the plane of collimation for the first set-up of the level is determined by adding the backsight to the reduced level of the bench mark. The reduced levels of the intermediate points and the first change point are then obtained by subtracting the staff readings taken on these points (I.S. and F.S.) from the elevation of the plane of collimation (H.I.). When the instrument is shifted to the second position, a new plane of collimation is set up. The levels of the two planes of collimation (first and second) are correlated by means of the backsight and foresight taken on the change point. The elevation of this plane is obtained by adding the new backsight taken on the change point from the second position of the level to the reduced level of the first change point. The elevation of this plane is obtained by adding the new backsight taken on the change point from the second position of the level to the reduced level of the first change point. The reduced levels of the successive points and the second change point are found by substracting their staff readings from the elevation of this plane of collimation. This process is repeated until all the reduced levels are worked out.

Arithmetic check = Σ B.S. – Σ F.S. = Last R.L. – First R.L.

(b)   The rise and fall system :

It consists in determining the difference of level between consecutive points by comparing each points after the first with that immediately proceeding it. The difference between their staff reading indicates a rise or a fall according as the staff reading at the point is smaller or greater that the proceeding point. The reduced level of each point is then found by adding the rise to, or substracting the fall from the reduced level of the preceding point.

Arithmetic check = Σ B.S. – Σ F.S. = Σ Rise – Σ Fall = Last R.L. – First R.S.

Observation Table and Results :

Staff Station	Reading			Rise	Fall	Height of instrument	Reduced level (R.L.)	Remarks
	Backsight	Intersight	Foresight					

Questions :

1. What is negative staff reading?
2. Which system is better : system of collimation or system of rise and fall?

Experiment No. 2

Object :

(a) To measure horizontal angle at a point by the method of repetition

(b) To measure horizontal angles at a point by the method of reiteration

Definitions of Terms :

    Centering : It means setting the theodolite over a station mark. It can be done by means of a plumb bob.

    Transiting (or plunging or reversing) : means the process of turning the telescope over its horizontal axis through 180° in a vertical plane.

    Face left (F.L.) : When vertical circle is on the left of the observer while taking a reading.

    Face right (F.R.) : When the vertical circle is on the right of the observer while taking a reading.

    Swinging the telescope : means turning the telescope in horizontal plane.

    Telescope normal : means "Bubble up" and Face left position.

    Changing face : means bringing the vertical circle to the right of the observer. It is originally to left and vice versa.

    Line of collimation (Line of sight) : It is the imaginary line joining the intersection of the cross hairs of the diaphragm to the optical centre of the object glass and its continuation.

    Axis of telescope : is the line joining the optical centre of the object glass to the centre of the eye piece.

    Axis of level tube (or Bubble line) : It is the straight line tangential to the longitudnal curve of the level tube at its centre.

    Vertical axis : is the axis about which the telescope can be rotated in a horizontal plane.

    Horizontal axis (Turnion axis) : It is the axis about which the telescope can be rotated in a vertical plane.

    Fundamental lines of a transit :

    (a) Vertical axis

    (b) Horizontal axis

    (c) Axis of altitude level tube

    (d) Axis of telescope

    (e) Line of collimation

Measurement of horizontal angles at a point by method of repetition

Procedure :

The procedure consists of :

    Making temporary adjustments :

    1. Set up the instrument and level it accurately. The face of instrument should be left and the telescope in the normal position.

    2. Release all clamps. Turn the upper plate till the zero of vernier A is against 0° of the main scale. Clamp the plates together. Bring 0° of vernier A to exactly over 0° of scale by the upper tangent screw.

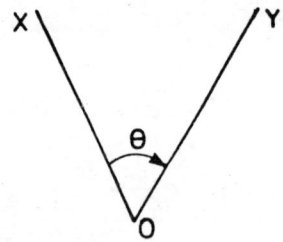 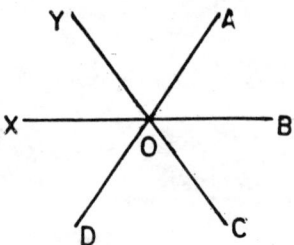

3. Loosen the lower clamp, direct the telescope to the left hand station (X) by using lower clamp and lower tangent screw.

4. Check the reading of vernier A to see that no slip has occured, and read the other vernier B. It should read 180° on the lower scale if there is no instrumental error.

5. Unclamp the upper (vernier) plate, turn the telescope *clockwise* and bisect the right-hand station (Y) exactly by using the upper clamp and upper slow motion screw.

6. Read both the verniers.

7. Leaving the verniers unchanged, unclamp the lower plate and turn the telescope clockwise until station X is again bisected accurately, using the lower clamp and lower tangent screw. Check the vernier readings which must be the same as before.

8. Release the upper plate, turn the telescope clockwise and again bisect the station Y exactly, using the upper clamp and its slow motion screw. The verniers will now read twice the value of the angle.

9. Repeat the process until the angle is repeated the required number of times (usually 3).

10. Read both verniers at the end the requisite repetition. Add 360° for every complete revolution to the final reading and divide the sum by the no. of repetitions. The result gives the correct value of XOY.

11. Change face (the telescope will now be inverted and the face will be right). Repeat the whole series of observations in exactly the same manner as for face left. The average of the two values of the angle thus obtained gives the value of angle XOY.

Conditions of permanent adjustments :

1. The axes of the plate levels must be perpendicular to the vertical axis.

2. The line of sight must be at right angles to the horizontal axis.

3. The horizontal axis must be perpendicular to the vertical axis.

4. When the instrument is levelled and the bubble attached to the vertical circle is central, the reading of the vertical circle should be zero or multiple of 90 degree.

Measurement of horizontal angles at a point by method of reiteration

Procedure :

In this method several angles are measured successively, and finally the horizon is closed, i.e. the angle between the last station and the initial station is measured. For measuring angles AOB, BOC, and COD proceed as follows :

1. Set up instrument over O and level it correctly.

2. Set the vernier A to zero.

3. Direct the telescope to point A and bisect it accurately by using the lower clamp and lower tangent screw. Note the vernier readings.

4. Loosen the upper plate and turn the telescope clockwise until point B is exactly bisected by turning

the upper tangent screw. Read both verniers. The mean of the verniers gives the value of angle AOB.

5. Similarly, bisect C and D successively, take readings of both verniers at each bisection.
6. Finally close the horizon by sighting the station point A.
7. The vernier A should now read 360 degree. If not, note the reading and find the error. If error is small, it is equally distributed among the several observed angles. If error is large, the readings should be discarded and a new set be taken.

Second set :

1. Change the face
2. Set the vernier A to 60 degrees or 90 degrees.
3. Again measure the angles in the same manner by turning the telescope this time in a counter clockwise direction to compensate for slip and errors due to twisting of the instrument. Bring the cross-hairs into exact coincidence with the stations from right to left, with upper, slow motion screw to eliminate the effects of backlash. Read both verniers at each bisection.
4. Further procedure is the same as in the first set.
5. The mean of the two sets is the true value of the angles.

Questions :

1. Why we take the readings on both the scales A and B?
2. Why we take the readings with face left and right?
3. Which error do you eliminate by method of repetition?

Observation Table for measuring horizontal angle at a point by method of repetition

Inst. Stn.	Object sighted	Face : Left			No. of Rept.	Swing : Left	Face : Right			No. of Rept.	Swing : Right	Average horz. angle
		A	B	Mean		Horz. angle	A	B	Mean		Horz. angle	
		° ′ ″	° ′ ″	° ′ ″		° ′ ″	° ′ ″	° ′ ″	° ′ ″		° ′ ″	

Observation Table for measurement of horizontal angles by method of reiteration

Inst. Stn.	Object sighted	Face : Left			Swing : Right	Face : Right			Swing : Left	Average horz. angle
		A	B	Mean	Horz. angle	A	B	Mean	Horz. angle	
		° ′ ″	° ′ ″	° ′ ″	° ′ ″	° ′ ″	° ′ ″	° ′ ″	° ′ ″	

Experiment No. 3

Object :

To determine the height of an object, the base of which is inaccessible.

Apparatus :

Theodolite, levelling staff, measuring tape, etc.

Procedure :

Two stations A and B are suitably chosen on a fairly level ground so as to lie in a vertical plane passing through the object (in line with object), and the distance between them is accurately measured. Then following steps have to be followed :

1. Set up the theodolite over station A. Having levelled it accurately, bisect the object.
2. With the vertical vernier reading zero, and with the altitude bubble central, take a reading on the staff held on B.M. or reference point.
3. Bisect the object and read both verniers. Take both face right and face left observations. Mean of four readings gives the correct value of the vertical angle.
4. Transit the theodolite and mark the second station B on the ground. Measure distance AB.
5. Shift the instrument to station B and take similar observations as at station A. From the vertical angles measurements and staff readings at the two stations and the distance between them, the vertical height can be found from the following trigonometrical relationships :

$$\frac{D}{h} = \cot \alpha_1 \qquad \qquad \text{...(i)}$$

$$\frac{D+b}{h+s} = \cot \alpha_2 \qquad \qquad \text{...(ii)}$$

$$\therefore \quad \frac{h \cot \alpha_1 + b}{h+s} = \cot \alpha_2$$

$$\text{or} \quad h = \frac{s \cot \alpha_2 - b}{\cot \alpha_1 - \cot \alpha_2} = \frac{(b + s \cot \alpha_2)(\tan \alpha_1)(\tan \alpha_2)}{\tan \alpha_1 - \tan \alpha_2}$$

$$H = (h + x)$$

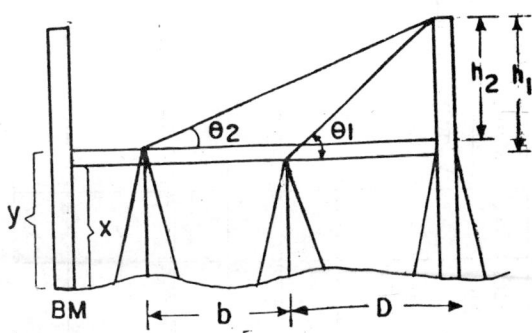

Similarly it can be shown that if B is lower than A, use (–) sign here. Use (+) sign if instrument axis at farther station is higher and (–) sign if instrument axis at the farther station is lower.

Observation Table :

Inst. Stn.	Object sighted	Face	Vertical Angle Reading			Angle	Mean angle	b	y	x	$s = y - x$	D	h (use formula)	$H = h + x$	Remarks
			Vernier C	Vernier D	Mean										
			° ′ ″	° ′ ″	° ′ ″	° ′ ″	° ′ ″								

Experiment No. 4

Object:

(a) To determine multiplying constant K and additive constant C of tacheometer.

(b) To find distance and elevations of five points around instrument station.

Procedure: (1)

1. Set out a line PQ about 100 to 150 meters long on a fairly level ground. fix pegs at 25 m interval.
2. Set up tacheometer at P and obtain the staff intercepts by taking stadia reading on staff held vertical on every point.
3. By substituting the values of different distances and staff intercepts in equation $D = KS + C$; a number of equations are obtained.
4. Solve these equations in pairs and obtain several sets of constants K and C. the mean of all the values are taken, to give constants K and C.

Procedure : (2)

1. Set the instrument at a point R
2. Record staff intercepts and angle of elevation or depression (if any) at five given points.
3. Calculate distances and elevations of there points for values of K and C as determined in procedure (1).

Observations :

Let elevation of instrument station R = 300 m

Height of instrument axis from ground = h =

Peg No.	Distance (m)	Staff Readings		$S = A - B$	$D = KS + C$	K	Av. K	C	Av. C
		Bottom A	Top B						
1	0								
2	25								
3	50								
4	75								
5	100								

(c) To find distances and elevations of five points around instrument station.

Staff station sighted	Staff Readings			Staff intercept $S = A - B$	Vertical Angle Reading			D	Elevation
	Bottom (A)	Centre (C)	Top (B)		Face Left	Face Right	Av.		
					° ′ ″	° ′ ″	° ′ ″		
P_1									
P_2									
P_3									
P_4									
P_5									

For calculating D and elevation, use appropriate expressions.

Questions :

1. Which is more accurate : tacheometer or theodolite?
2. Can we use theodolite as a tacheometer? If yes, how?

Experiment No. 5

Object :

To determine the height of a tall object by two plane method.

Apparatus :

Theodolite, staff, tape, peg, etc.

Theory :

From Figure,

Δ QRQ′

$Q'Q = h_1 = RQ' \tan \alpha_1$

Δ PQQ″

$QQ'' = h_2 = PQ'' \tan \alpha_2$

QRQ′ and PQQ″ are vertical triangles

Applying sine rule

$$\frac{\sin \theta_2}{AQ_1} = \frac{\sin \theta_1}{BQ_1} = \frac{\sin [\pi - (\theta_1 + \theta_2)]}{AB}$$

$AQ_1 = RQ'$, $BQ_1 = PQ''$, $AB = PR = d$

$$\frac{\sin \theta_2}{RQ'} = \frac{\sin (\theta_1 + \theta_2)}{d}$$

$$RQ' = d \, \frac{\sin \theta_2}{\sin (\theta_1 + \theta_2)}$$

$$\frac{\sin \theta_1}{PQ''} = \frac{\sin (\theta_1 + \theta_2)}{d}$$

$$PQ'' = \frac{d \sin \theta_1}{\sin (\theta_1 + \theta_2)}$$

$\therefore$ RL of Q = RL of BM + ht. of instrument + h_1 (at A) ...(1a)

RL of Q = RL of BM + ht. of instrument + h_2 (at B) ...(1b)

$$h_1 = \frac{d (\tan \theta_1 \sin \theta_2)}{\sin (\theta_1 + \theta_2)}, \qquad h_2 = \frac{d \sin \theta_1 \tan \theta_2}{\sin (\theta_1 + \theta_2)}$$

Procedure :

1. Set the theodolite at station A, level it and drive a peg at A into the ground. Set the zero reading on horizontal scale and sight the object. Image of the object should lie on vertical cross hair.
2. Sight the top of the object by rotating the vertical main scale, and measure the angle of elevation α_1.
3. Now sight the second instrument station and measure the horizontal angle θ_1.

4. Set the zero reading on the vertical scale and sight the staff which is placed on B.M. and determine the height of instrument at A.

5. Shift the theodolite to another station B. Level it and similarly measure α_2, θ_2 and height of instrument at B. Measure the distance 'd' between the two stations.

Observations :

$\theta_1 =$

$\theta_2 =$

$\alpha_1 =$

$\alpha_2 =$

$d =$

Ht. of instrument at A =

Ht. of instrument at B =

RL of BM =

Calculation :

Put the values in formula (1a) or (1b) and determine the RL of object.

Result :

RL of object =

RL of BM =

Ht. of object =

Questions :

1. Which method is better : one plane method or two plane method?
2. When should we go for two plane method?

Experiment No. 6

Object :

Profile levelling of a path.

Apparatus :

Level, chain, tape, arrows, etc.

Theory :

Profile levelling or longitudinal sectioning is the process of determining the elevations of points along the centre line of canals, sewer, highway, etc. It enables the engineers to study the relationship between the existing ground surface and the levels of the proposed construction in the direction of centre line.

Procedure :

1. Set out the centre line. Along the centre line at fixed interval, select some points and draw the perpendicular through each point of centre line and place some pegs on each of these perpendiculars.
2. Select a point for instrument station and set the level.
3. Put the staff at B.M. Note the staff reading and determine the height of instrument.
4. Put the staff at a point which is on perpendicular drawn earlier and take the staff reading.
5. Similarly take the staff readings for all those points which can be seen easily and clearly from this instrument station.
6. Now shift the level to some other point and determine the height of instrument.
7. Take the staff readings for all clearly visible points and determine their elevations.
8. Repeat step (6) and (7) until the whole site is surveyed.
9. Plot the profile of centre line and perpendicular line on graph papers.

Observations :

Station	BS	IS	FS	HI	RL	Remarks
BM						
1						
2						
1						
T_p						
1						
1						
T_p						
1						

Result :

The profiles are plotted on graph papers.

Precaution :

When the vertical profile of the ground is regular or gradually curving, readings should be taken on points at fixed interval. If irregular ground or abrupt changes of slope occur the interval chosen should be small.

   (T_p = turning point)

Experiment No. 7

Object :

Chain and theodolite traversing (close traversing).

Apparatus :

Theodolite fitted with compass, tape, chain, ranging rods, etc.

Theory :

In traverse surveying the number of connected lines are surveyed. If these lines form a closed loop then it is called closed traversing otherwise open traversing. Closed traverse is used for locating the boundaries of lakes, woods, buildings, etc., and open traversing is suitable for highway, canal surveying, etc.

Procedure :

1. Set the theodolite at station A. Set the zero reading on horizontal scale of theodolite. Loose the clamp of the magnetic needle. Using lower clamp and tangent screw point the telescope to magnetic meridian.
2. Loosen the upper clamp and rotate the telescope and sight the other station B. Take the reading which gives the magnetic bearing of the line AB.
3. Spread the chain between stations A and B. If the chain is shorter than length of AB then ranging must be done.
4. Measure the offsets of details adjacent to chain. (Offsets should be taken in order of their chainage).
5. Take the offsets and chain length for all the details between the two stations A and B.
6. Shift the theodolite to point B. Sight other station C. Measure the included angle subtended by AB and BC at B.
7. Repeat the steps 3 to 5 to survey the details adjacent to chain line BC.
8. Shift the theodolite to point C. Sight the other station D. Measure the included angle BCD and survey all the details as explained earlier.
9. Repeat this process until the point A is reached.

Observations :

Magnetic Bearing of line AB =

Angle	Vernier Reading	Magnetic Bearing
∠ABC		line BC
∠BCD		line CD
Offset Readings :		

ΔA
.
.
.
ΔB
.
.
.
ΔA

Result :

Plot the details of given area.

Experiment No. 8

Object :

Triangulation survey.

Apparatus :

Steel tape, theodolite, spring balance, thermometer, staff, pegs, etc.

Theory :

Triangulation is the system of inter connected triangles. In this system the length of only one line called base line and two among the three angles of the triangles are measured. Knowing the one side and the two angles the length of other two sides of triangle can be computed.

The length of base line is measured by steel tape. Various corrections are applied to measured length and finally corrected length is achieved. The corrections are as follows.

1. Correction for standardization (R) :

$$C_a = \frac{L.C}{l}$$

C_a = correction for absolute length

L = measured length of line

l = designated length of chain

C = correction per chain length

C_a will be positive if l < actual length of chain otherwise it will be negative.

2. Correction for slope :

$$C = L - \sqrt{L^2 - h^2}$$

L = measured length

h = difference in elevation at the two ends of line

C is always negative.

3. Correction for temperature :

$$L_t = \alpha \, (T_m - T_o) \, L$$

α = coefficient of thermal expansion

T_m = temperature (mean) of field

T_o = standard temperature

L = measured length

4. Correction for pull or tension :

$$C_p = \frac{P - P_o}{AE} L$$

P = applied pull during measurement

P_o = standard pull

L = measured length

A = cross sectional area of the tape

E = Young's modules of elasticity.

5. *Correction for sag :*

$$CS_1 = \frac{l_i (Wl_i)^2}{24 p^2}$$

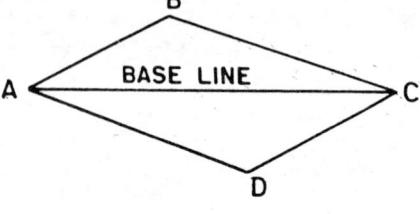

l_i = length of tape suspended between the supports

P = applied pull

W = wt. of tape per unit length.

Procedure :

1. Drive a peg on each vertex of the triangles
2. Set the theodolite at station A and measure the angles $\angle DAC$ and $\angle CAB$ precisely.
3. Shift the theodolite to point C and measure the angles $\angle DCA$ and $\angle ACB$.
4. Measure the length of the tape at some standard gauge. Note down the field temperature also.
5. Generally the length of base line is greater than a tape length so drive some pegs on AC.
6. Attach the spring balance at the end of the tape with arrow at C and pull the tape. Note down the pull and staff readings at both ends of the tape by theodolite.
7. Repeat the step (6) until the station A is reached.
8. For more accuracy, now start from A and measure the length of AC.
9. Apply the corrections and find out the corrected base line length.

Observations :

$\angle DAC$ =

$\angle CAB$ =

$\angle DCA$ =

$\angle BCA$ =

Measured	Pull	Elevation Difference	Temperature
L_1			
L_2			
L_3			
L_4			
L_5			

Length	C_a	C_s	C_t	C_p	Sag	Total correction	Corrected length
L_1							
L_2							
L_3							
L_4							
L_5							

Calculations :

Total correction $= \pm C_a - C_s \pm C_t \pm C_p - \text{sag}$

Total corrected length $= \Sigma$ corrected lengths. Apply the sine rule and determine the length of DA, DC, AB, BC.

Result :

	Measured length	Theoretical lengths
DA		
DC		
AB		
BC		

Questions :

1. Why some corrections are both, i.e., positive and negative?
2. How the corrections have signs?

Experiment No. 9

Object :

Plotting the details of given area by plane table.

Apparatus :

Plane table, alidade, compass, level, plumbing fork, tape, drawing sheets, ranging rods.

Theory :

It is a graphical method of survey in which observations of fields and plotting of them simultaneously. Generally radiation and intersection methods are used in plotting the details.

Radiation : A ray is drawn from instrument station in the direction of object (point). The distance in between the instrument station and object is measured and by adopting a suitable scale a point is marked on the ray.

Intersection : A point corresponding to an object is plotted by intersection of two rays drawn from two different instrument stations in the direction of object.

Procedure :

1. Set the table at some place. Level the table and drive a peg in the ground. Now clamp the board and attach a sheet on the board. Transfer the point corresponding to peg (instrument station) on the sheet by plumbing fork. Insert a pin at this point on the board.

2. Draw a magnetic North-South line by compass. It will be helpful in orienting the table on another station.

3. Keep the alidade in touch with the pin (at instrument station point) and sight a point. Draw a line along the working edge of alidade. Measure the distance between the instrument station and point and mark a point on drawn line by taking a suitable scale. Similarly sight other points and draw the lines. Measure their distances from instrument station and plot them on the corresponding lines.

4. Now sight those point whose distances from the instrument station cannot be measured. Draw the lines from instrument station in their corresponding direction. Mark some identifying symbol or letter on these lines to avoid confusion. These point will be plotted by intersection method.

5. Select a second instrument station, sight it from station A and draw a line in this direction. Measure the distance between two stations and plot it on sheet with same scale.

6. Transfer the table on second instrument station.

7. Level and orient the table to achieve the correct centering of table. Orientation must be done by compass as well as by back sighting.

8. Now sight all those point which are to be plotted by intersection method. Draw the lines in respective directions from instrument station. The intersection of two lines for point from different stations gives the location of that point on sheet. In this way find out all such point by intersection.

9. Plot all those points also whose distances can be measured from this station.

Result :

Detail of area has been plotted on sheet.

Precaution :

1. While orienting the table by compass there should not be such type of material nearby which deviated the compass needle.
2. Always use the fictitious edge of alidade in drawing the line.

Questions :

1. When should we go for intersection method?
2. When is the method of radiation useful?

Experiment No. 10

Object :

Determine the position of an instrument station.

Apparatus :

Plane table, plumbing fork, level, compass, etc.

Theory :

Position of instrument station is determined by observing three points whose position have been previously plotted on sheet. It is called three points problem. The table is oriented by trial and error. Therefore it is also called trial and error method or Lehman's method.

Lehman Rule : If the station is outside the great triangle (whose vertices are three plotted point) the error triangle will also fall outside the great triangle. Similarly if the station is inside the great triangle the error triangle will also be inside the great triangle and point should be chosen inside the error triangle.

The point should be so chosen that its distance from the rays, Aa, Bb, Cc (as shown in figure) is proportional to the distance of station from A, B, C points respectively and it should be on the same side of all three rays.

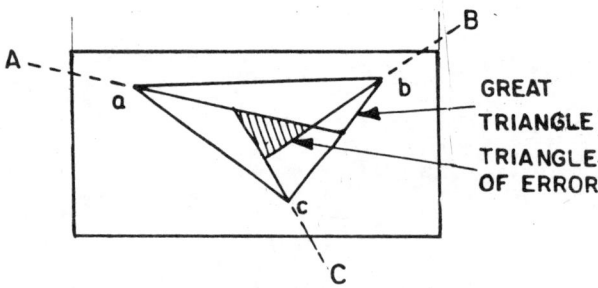

Procedure :

1. Set the table at the station P and orient the table approximately so that ab is parallel to AB and clamp the table.
2. Keep the alidade pivoted about a and sight A. Draw the ray. Similarly, draw rays from b and c towards B and C respectively. If the orientation is correct, the three rays will meet at one point. If not, they will meet at three points forming one small triangle of error.
3. The triangle of error so formed will give the idea for further orientation. The orientation will be correct only when the triangle of error is reduced to a point. The approximate choice of the position will be done with the help of Lehman's Rules.
4. Keep the alidade along A and rotate the table to sight A and clamp the table. This will give next approximate orientation (but more accurate than the previous one).

5. Keep the alidade at b to sight B and draw the ray. Similarly, keep the alidade at c and sight C. Draw the ray. These rays will again form a triangle in case orientation is not perfect but the size of which will be smaller than the previous triangle (if p′ has been chosen intelligently keeping in view the Lehman's Rules).

6. Thus, by successive trial and error, the triangle of error can be reduced to a point. The final and correct position of the table will be such that the rays Aa, and Cc meet at one single point, giving the point p.

Result :

The position of the station determined.

Precaution :

1. Choose the point by following the Lehman rule otherwise size of error triangle may be increased.

Question :

1. What will happen if all three points and instrument station lie on a circle?

Experiment No. 11

Object :

Contour survey of a given area using square method.

Apparatus :

Level, staff, chain, tape, pegs, etc.

Theory :

In the square method of contour surveying, the elevation for some guide points are found. Contours of a desired elevation is plotted by linear interpolation. These guide points lie on the vertices of square or rectangles on the ground.

Procedure :

1. Divide the area into a number of squares by chain and tape. The size of square depends upon the size of ground to be surveyed. Drive the pegs on the corners of the squares.
2. Fix the level in the middle of the area.
3. Find elevations of corners of squares by means of level and staff.
4. Plot the contours of various elevations by linear interpolation which implies the uniform slope between two points.

Limitation :

It is used when ground is not much undulating and the given area is small.

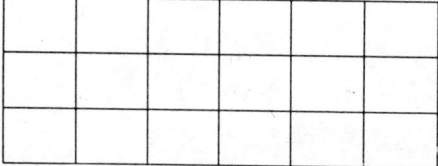

Observation Table :

R.L. of bench mark =
Staff reading at bench mark =
Height of instrument =

Staff station		Staff reading	Elevation of the point
a	1		
	2		
	3		
	4		
b	1		
	2		
	3		
	4		
c	1		
	2		
	3		
	4		

Questions :

1. What are the different advantages of square method?
2. What do you understand by contouring?

Experiment No. 12

Object :

Contour surveying by tacheometric method.

Apparatus :

Tacheometer, staff, etc.

Theory :

A tacheometer is a theodolite fitted with static diaphragm so that staff readings against all the three hairs may be taken. The staff intercept which is vertical distance between top and bottom hair on the staff image is determined. After determining the staff intercept there is no need to measure the horizontal distance since tacheometer controls both horizontal and vertical distances.

Tacheometer formula.

$$D = K_1 S \cos^2 \theta + K_2 \cos \theta \qquad \qquad ...(i)$$
$$V = D \tan \theta \qquad \qquad ...(ii)$$

where D = horizontal distance between instrument and staff

S = Staff intercept

V = vertical difference in elevation between the instrument axis and the point in which the line of sight against the central wire intersects the staff.

θ = Inclination of line of sight with horizontal.

K_1 and K_2 are tacheometric constants.

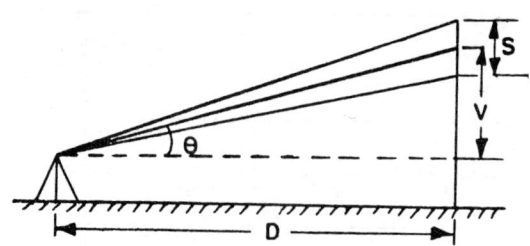

Procedure :

(a) To determine the tacheometric constants.

1. Set the tacheometer in plain ground.
2. Sight the staff placed at a point and find out the staff intercept(s) for that point.
3. Measure the horizontal distance between staff and tacheometer (D). Set the zero on vertical scale of tacheometer, i.e., $\theta = 0$.
4. Repeat the step (2) and (3) for another point and determine D and S for this point also.

For $\theta = 0$

$$D = K_1 S + K_2 \qquad\qquad \text{...(ia)}$$

From two sets of D and S values determine the K_1 and K_2 by equation (ia).

(b) Contour surveying to determine the height of instrument.

1. Shift the instrument to the area which is to be surveyed and set the instrument at convenient place.
2. Set the zero reading on horizontal scale.
3. Sight the staff and determine the staff reading. If necessary, set any angle on vertical scale also and note it.
4. Without changing the horizontal scale position of instrument, shift the staff to another point and determine the staff intercept and vertical angle also. Take five to six such readings for a fixed horizontal reading. Thus the survey along one radial line is over.
5. Set up another angle on horizontal scale and repeat the steps (3) and (4).
6. Like this, survey the whole area in 5 to 6 radial lines and plot the contours.

Observation :

R.L. of bench mark =

Staff reading at bench mark against mid hair (when $\theta = 0$) =

Ht. of instruments =

Calculations :

Determine value of K_1 and K_2 from equation (ia).

Determine D and V for each staff station from equations (i) and (ii).

Radial position		1	2	3	4	5	6
0°	Top reading						
	Mid reading						
	Bottom reading						
	Staff interception						
	Vertical angle						
	D =						
	V =						
60°	Top reading						
	Mid reading						
	Bottom reading						
	Staff interception						
	Vertical angle						
	D =						
	V =						

Result :

Contours have been plotted for given area.

$K_1 =$

$K_2 =$

Limitation :

Tacheometric method is used in hilly areas.

Experiment No. 13

Object :

To trace out the simple circular curve with the help of chain and tape only.

Apparatus :

Chain, tape, arrows, pegs, etc.

Theory :

Let $A_1T_1 = AT_1 =$ initial chord C_1

T_1V is the rear tangent at T_1.

$\angle A_1T_1A$ is deflection angle of first chord $= \delta$

From geometry

Arc $A_1A = AT_1 \delta$ (chord)   (δ is in radian)   ...(i)

In triangle AT_1A'

$$A'T_1 = A'A$$

$\therefore$ $\angle A'T_1A = AAT_1 = \delta$

In triangle AT_1O

$OT_1 = OA =$ radius of circle

$\angle OT_1A = \angle OAT_1$

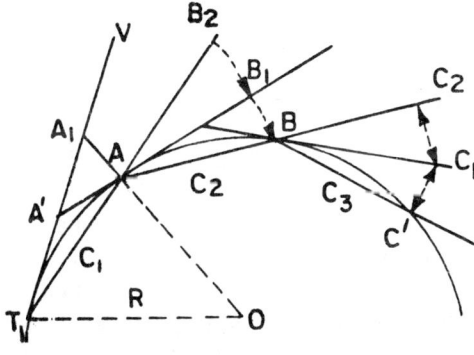

$\angle OT_1A = \angle OT_1A' - \angle AT_1A$ $\because$ $\angle OT_1A = 90°$

$= 90° - \delta$ (angle between tangent and radius)

Therefore $\angle T_1OA = 180° - 2(90° - \delta)$

$= 2\delta$.

Arc $T_1A = T_1O (2\delta)$

$= R (2\delta)$, $R =$ radius of circle.

$\therefore$ $\delta = \dfrac{T_1A}{2R}$ ...(ii)

From (i) and (ii),

$$A_1A = \dfrac{AT_1 . T_1A}{2R}$$

Assuming arc $T_1A =$ chord $AT_1 = C_1 =$ initial chord.

$A_1A =$ first offset $= \dfrac{C_1^2}{2R}$ ...(iii)

For second offset B_2B

AB_1 is tangent at A

As shown in eqn. (iii),

The offset from tangent $= B_1B = \dfrac{C_2^2}{2R}$

$\angle B_2AB_1 = A'AT_1$ opposite angles

$\qquad = \delta$

$\therefore$ Arc $B_2B_1 = AB_2\delta$

$\qquad\qquad = \dfrac{C_2^2}{2R}$

Off set $B_22B = B_2B_1 + B_1B.$

$\qquad = \dfrac{C_2^2}{2R} + \dfrac{C_1\,C_2}{2R}$

$\qquad = \dfrac{C_2}{2R}(C_1 + C_2)$

like this for nth point.

Offset from $(n-1)$th point produced chord

$\qquad = \dfrac{C_n}{2R}(C_n + C_n - 1)$

If first chord is of length C

last chord is of C'

and all intermediate chords $= C$

then $C_1 = \dfrac{C_2}{2R}$

$C_2 = \dfrac{(C+C)}{2R}$

$C_3 = C_4 = C_n - 1 = \dfrac{C^2}{2R}$

$C_n = C \text{ last} = \dfrac{C'(C+C')}{2R}$

From the simple geometry for any simple circular curve.

tangent length $= VT_1 = VT_2 = R \tan \Delta/2$ (from $\triangle VT_1O$)

chord length $T_1T_2 = 2R \sin \Delta/2$ (from $\triangle T_1OC$)

length of curve $T_1T_2 = R\Delta.$

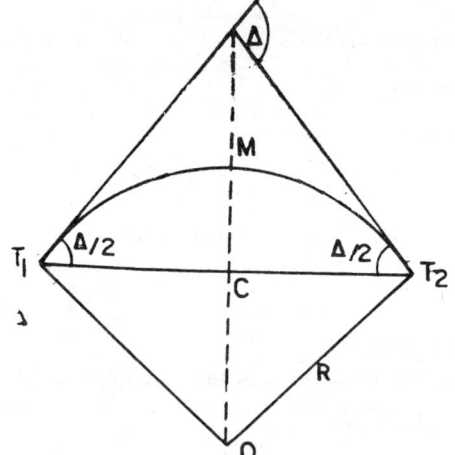

Data Given :

Radius of curve $= R$

Angle of Intersection $= \Delta$

Chainage of point of Intersection

Procedure :

First calculate the tangent length. Determine the chainage of point T_1 and T_2.

Chainage of point T_1 = chainage of point of intersection – tangent length

Chainage of point T_2 = chainage of point T_1 + curve length T_1T_2

Decide the length of normal chord. Generally the length is taken ten or twenty metre.

Determine the length of first chord. The length of first chord and last chord are always less than the length of normal. Chord length of first chord is fixed in such a way that chainage of first point on the curve (point A in the figure) is multiple of normal chord. Similarly, the last chord length is determined in such a way that chainage of last but one point (prior to point T_2) is multiple of normal chord.

1. Locate point T_1 on the ground and spread the chain or tape with its one end at T_1 in the direction of rear tangent to the point A_1 such that $T_1A_1 = C =$ length of first chord.

2. With T_1 as centre and T_1A_1 as radius, swing the chain such that $A_1A =$ first offset, O_1. Fix the point A by driving the peg in the ground.

3. Spread the chain straight along $T'A$ and pull it straight in the direction such that its zero is at A. With zero of chain at A and radius $OB_2 = C =$ length of normal chord. Swing the chain such that $B_2B =$ second offset O_2. Fix the point B.

4. Spread the chain along AB and repeat the step (3) until the last point T_2 is reached.

5. After getting point T_2 measure the length (straight) of T_1T_2 and compare it with calculated value of chord length.

Calculation :

Length of chord (T_1T_2) (calculated) =
Length of curve =
Chainage of point of intersection =
Chainage of point T_1 =
Chainage of point T_2 =

Result :

Calculated length of T_1T_2 =
Measured length T_1T_2 =

Precaution :

Apply the proper pull to spread the chain straight, i.e., chain must be straight while measuring the length.

Limitation :

It is not very accurate method.

Question :

What is the advantage of setting the curve by tape and chain?

Experiment No. 14

Object :

To trace out a simple circular curve by theodolite.

Apparatus :

Theodolite, pegs, rods, tape, etc.

Theory :

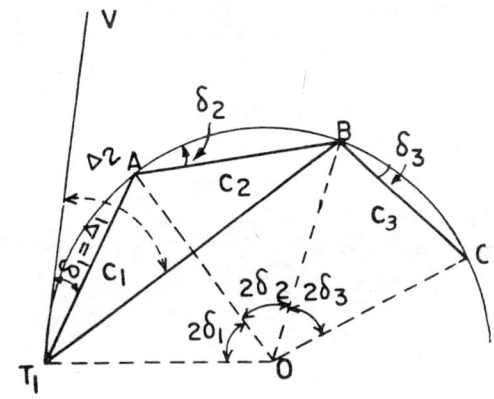

T_1V = rear tangent

δ_i = tangential angles

O_i = total tangential angle

C_i's = length of chord.

From simple geometry :

Assuming arc T_1A = chord $T_1A = C_1$

$$\therefore \quad \frac{C_1}{2\,\delta_1} = \frac{\pi R}{180} \quad \text{where } \delta_1 \text{ is in degrees.}$$

For first chord $\delta_1 = \Delta_1$ as shown in figure.

Therefore, $\Delta_1 = \dfrac{90\,C_1}{\pi R}$ in degrees

$$= 1718.9\,\frac{C_1}{R} \text{ in minutes.}$$

Similarly $\delta_i = \dfrac{1718.9\,C_i}{R}$

From figure $\Delta_2 = \angle A_1T_1A + \angle AT_1B = \angle A_1T_1B = \angle VT_1B$

$$\Delta_2 = \delta_1 + \frac{1}{2}\angle AOB = \delta_1 + 2 \times \frac{1}{2}\delta_2$$

$$= \delta_1 + \delta_2$$

Since $\angle AT_1B = 1/2\,\angle AOB$ (angle subtended by any arc at circumference is half of that subtended at centre of curve)

$$\Delta_2 = \delta_1 + \delta_2$$

$$\Delta_3 = \delta_1 + \delta_2 + \delta_3$$

$$\Delta_i = \delta_1 + \ldots \ldots + \delta_i$$

Procedure :

Calculate the tangent length, curve length, chord length and subchords, normal chords from given data.

1. Locate the point of intersection and from this point locate the point of curve, i.e., T_1 in a fixed direction at a distance of tangent length. Fix a rod with flag at the point of intersection.

2. Set the theodolite at T_1. Direct the theodolite to bisect the point of intersection. Thus line of sight is in the direction of rear tangent. Clamp both the plates of theodolite at zero reading.

3. Release the upper plate of theodolite, i.e., vernier plate and set an angle Δ_1. Hold the zero of the tape at point T_1. Take the length of first chord on tape and on this mark of tape, attach an arrow. Now swing the tape with radius as first chord length and centre at T_1 until the arrow is bisected by the cross hairs. Thus the first point A is fixed. Drive a peg into the ground at this point.

4. Set the Δ_2 on theodolite. Now take the length of second chord on tape, hold the zero of tape at A and swing it until the arrow is bisected by cross hair and get the point B.

5. Repeat the step (4) until the last point is reached.

Check :

Measure the chord length (T_1T_2) and tangent length VT_2 and compare them with calculated values respectively.

Observation :

Point chainage	Chord length (C)	Tangential angle	Total tangential angle	Actual theodolite reading

Result :

Measured tangent length (VT_2) =
Calculated tangent length =
Calculated chord length =
Measured chord length =

Precaution :

Angle should be set by fine screw to avoid the error in setting the angle.

Experiment No. 15

Object :

To trace out the compound curve.

Apparatus :

Theodolite, tape, chain, peg, etc.

Theory :

From figure,

$$t_s = T_1 D_1 = R_S \tan (\tfrac{1}{2} \Delta_1) \qquad \text{...(ia)}$$

$$t_L = R_L \tan (\tfrac{1}{2} \Delta_2) \qquad \text{...(ib)}$$

$$\Delta = \Delta_1 + \Delta_2$$

From triangle VT_1T_2

$$\frac{D_1 V}{D_1 D_2} = \frac{\sin \Delta_2}{\sin \Delta}$$

$$D_1 V = (t_s + t_l) \frac{\sin \Delta_2}{\sin \Delta}$$

$$\frac{D_2 V}{D_1 D_2} = \frac{\sin \Delta_1}{\sin \Delta}$$

$$D_2 V = (t_s + t_l) \frac{\sin \Delta_1}{\sin \Delta}$$

$$T_s = t_s + D_1 V = R_S \tan (\tfrac{1}{2} \Delta_1) + (t_S + t_L) \frac{\sin \Delta_2}{\sin \Delta}$$

$$T_L = t_L + D_2 V = t_L + (t_S + t_L) \frac{\sin \Delta_1}{\sin \Delta}$$

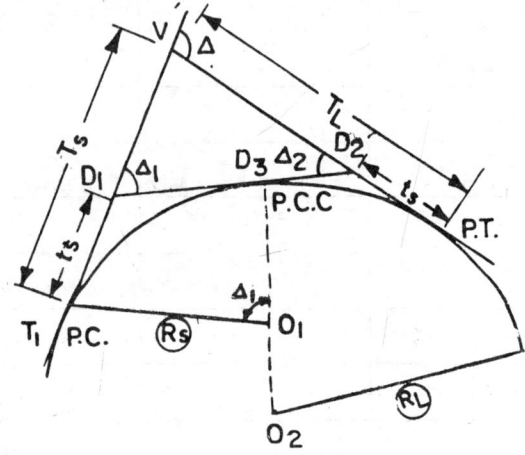

Data given :

Δ, R_L, R_S, Δ_2 (or Δ_1)
Required Δ_1 (or Δ_2), T_S, T_L.

Procedure :

1. By knowing the four quantities (given data) determine the rest three quantities by developed formulae.
2. Select the point of intersection (V) and by measuring appropriate tangent length find the point T_1, i.e., point of curve.
3. Set the theodolite at T_1 and sight the point of intersection with zero reading on horizontal scale.
4. Calculate the length of curves and by knowing the chainage of V, determine the chainage of T_1, D_3, T_2. Calculate the length of sub-chords also.

5. By length of chords determine the Δ_i's for both curves.
6. Set the angle Δ_i's on the horizontal scale and set out the first branch of the curve by Rankine method.
7. After locating the P.C.C. shift the theodolite to P.C.C. (i.e., point D_3) and set the theodolite there.
8. Backsight the point T_1 with the horizontal reading $(360 - \Delta_1/2)$.
9. By setting the Δ_i's for second curve set out the second branch of the curve from D_3 until T_2 is reached.
10. Check the observations by measuring the angle $T_1D_3T_2$ which should be equal to $(180 - \Delta/2)$.

Observations :

Chainage of P.I. =

T_S =   Chainage of P.C. =

L_S =   Chainage of P.C.C. =

t_1 =   Chainage of P.T. =

Chord length for first curve

C_1 = C_2 = C_3 = ...$C_n - 1$ = C_n =

Chord length for second curve

C_1 = C_2 = C_3 = ...$C_n - 1$ = C_n =

Observation Table :

Point Chainage	Chord length	Tangential angle δ_i	Deflector angle Δ_1	Actual theodolite reading

Similarly for another branch of curve.

$$\delta_i = 1718.9 \frac{C_i}{R} \text{ minutes}$$

$$\Delta_i = \sum_{i=1}^{i=i} \delta_i$$

R may be R_S or R_L depending upon branch of curve

$\angle T_1D_3T_2 =$

Calculations :

Given, Δ, R_L, R_S, Δ_2 and chainage of P.I.

$\Delta_1 = \Delta - \Delta_2$ $\angle T_1 D_3 T_2 = 180 - \Delta / 2$

$$T_S = t_s + (t_s + t_l) \frac{\sin \Delta_2}{\sin \Delta}$$

$$T_L = t_i + (t_s + t_L) \frac{\sin \Delta_1}{\sin \Delta}$$

$t_s = R_S \tan (\frac{1}{2} \Delta_1)$

$t_L = R_L \tan (\frac{1}{2} \Delta_2)$

$1l = R_L \Delta_2$ (Δ_2 in radians)

$1s = R_S \Delta_1$ (Δ_1 in radians)

Result :

The compound curve has been traced out.

Observed $\angle T_1 D_3 T_2 =$

Theoretical $\angle T_1 D_3 T_2 =$

Questions :

1. Define different types of curves.
2. What are the main differences in tracing out these curves?

Experiment No. 16

Object :

To trace out the Bernoulli's lemniscate curve.

Apparatus :

Theodolite, peg, tape, etc.

Theory :

The polar equation of Bernoulli's lemniscate is

$b = k \sqrt{\sin 2\alpha}$

The deviation angle ϕ is three times the polar deflection angle (α) for lemniscate curve.

$\phi = 3\alpha$

From the geometry of figure,

$\angle AVC = \frac{1}{2}(180 - \Delta) = 90 - \Delta/2$

$\therefore \quad \angle VAC = 180 - (90 - \Delta/2 + 90) = \Delta/2 = \phi$

$\phi/3 = \alpha = \Delta/6$

From the triangle $\Delta\ T_1AC$

$$\frac{T_1V}{\sin(\angle T_1CV)} = \frac{VC}{\sin(\angle VT_1C)}$$

$\angle T_1CV = 180 - (90 - \Delta/2) - \alpha$

$\qquad = 90 + \Delta/2 - \Delta/6$

$\qquad = 90 + \dfrac{\Delta}{3}$

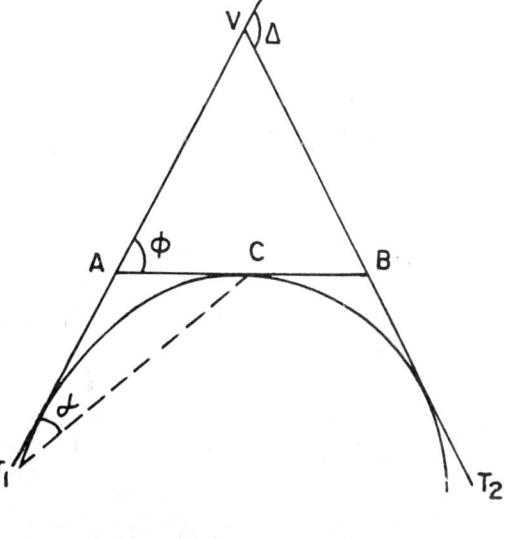

Data given :

Apex distance VC, angle of intersection $\angle\ T_1VT_2$.

$$\therefore \quad \frac{T_1V}{\sin(90 + \Delta/3)} = \frac{VC}{\sin(\Delta/6)}$$

$$T_1V = \frac{\cos \Delta/3}{\sin \Delta/6}\ VC$$

$$\frac{T_1C}{\sin(90 - \Delta/2)} = \frac{VC}{\sin \alpha}$$

$$T_1C = VC\ \frac{\cos \Delta/2}{\sin \Delta/6}$$

Procedure :

1. Select the point of intersection. By measuring the tangential length T_1V, find the P.C., i.e., T_1.

2. Set the theodolite at T_1. Sight P.I. while there is zero reading on horizontal scale.

3. Set the first deflection angle (α_1) at the theodolite and measure the distance b_1 along the line of sight. Find the first point on the curve and insert a peg into the ground.

4. Similarly find other points on the curve until the point C is set out. For all the points measure the chord length from the point T_1.

5. To set out the other half, shift the theodolite to the point T_2 and repeat the procedure as earlier until the point C is set out.

Observations :

α	
b	

VC =

Calculations :

Δ and VC are given.

Tangent length $T_1V = \dfrac{\cos \Delta/3}{\sin \Delta/6} VC$

Final chord, i.e., $b_n = T_1C = \dfrac{\cos \Delta/2}{\sin \Delta/6} VC$

Final deflection angle $\alpha_n = \alpha = \Delta/6$

$K = \dfrac{b_n}{\sqrt{\sin 2\alpha_n}}$

Result :

Bernoulli's lemniscate has been traced out.

Given apex distance VC =

Measured apex distance VC =

Experiment No. 17

Object :

To study the minor instruments.

a) Open Cross Staff :

It is used for setting out sight angles. It consists of two pairs of vertical slits forming two line of sights at right angle to each other. The cross staff is set up at the point on the line from which right angle to be seen. Then it is turned until the ranging rod on survey line is visible through a pair of slits. The line of sight through other pair of slits will be at right angle to survey line at the staff point and ranging rod may be established in this direction.

b) French Cross Staff :

It is provided with a hollow octagonal box. In middle of each face of the box vertical slits are cut through them object is sighted. By the french cross staff the angle of 45° or 90° can be set out.

c) Adjustable Cross Staff

This staff consists of two cylinders of equal diameter placed one on the top of other. Both the cylinders are provided with sighting slits. The upper one can be rotated relative to lower cylinder by some arrangement. The upper cylinder carries a vernier also. The lower cylinder is graduated to degrees and subdivisions. This instrument enables the user to set out any angle.

d) Optical Square :

Optical square is a circular box with three slits A, B and C. A glass silvered at the top and unsilvered at the bottom is fixed in the line passing through A and C. An another glass is fixed at an angle of 45° to the previous glass facing to the slit B.

Any ray from the object in the slit C passes through the lower unsilvered portion of the mirror and reached to eye through slit A. Another ray from object in slit b side reflects the facing mirror and approaches to another mirror. Here it is again reflected and in such away that after reflection it reaches to eye after passing through the slit. A. Thus the objects which are at right angle can be seen in the same vertical line.

If one has to set a right angle on a survey line then the instrument is held on the line on the point at which perpendicular is to run. The slits A and C are directed towards the ranging rod on survey line. Then these very or directs the perpendicular to the survey line, to move till the two images coincide.

e) Ceylon Ghat Tracer :

It is used to setting out the gradients and to measure the slopes. It consists of circular tube with a peep hole at one end and cross wire at other end. Tube is supported by a 'A' frame with a hole at its top. This hole is used to fix the instrument to a stand. A heavy weight slides along the tube by some arrangement. The tube is engraved to give the readings of gradient. When the weight is against zero reading the line of sight is horizontal. For measuring the slope of line, (ground), the instrument is hold at one end and the target is hold at the another end. Target is having a circular spot which is sighted through the instrument. After the adjustment of line of sight by sliding the weight along the tube the circular spot is sighted and value of gradient is directly read from the engraved scale on the tube.

f) Box Sextant :

It is used for measuring the horizontal and vertical angle. It consists of a circular box of 8 cm in diameter and 4 cm in height. There are two glasses in the box. One is fixed and another is movable. The fixed horizontal glass is silvered at the lower half and plain at the upper half and the movable index glass is fully silvered. An index arm is pivoted at the index glass and carries a vernier.

Measurement of Angle by Box Sextant :

Instrument is held in the right hand and is brought into the plane of the eye and two points are observed. Left hand object is sighted through the eye hole and lower unsilvered portion of the horizon glass.

Hand Level :

It consists of rectangular or circular tube 10 to 15 cm long provided with a small bubble tube at the top. The line of sight passes through a pin hole at the eye end and a horizontal wire at the object end. A mirror is provided at 45° to the axis below the bubble tube by which the bubble can be seen at the instant of object is sighted. The mirror occupies only half the width of the tube and the object sighted through the other half. The line of sight is horizontal when the bubble appears opposite the cross wire. If it is not then it is made by rising or lowering the object end of level and reading is observed. As it is clear from its name it is held in the hand while used. It is used in locating the contours on the ground and also for short cross sectioning.

Abhey Level :

It is provided with a square tube with the peep hole at the one end and the cross wire at the another. The line passing through them is called line of sight. A mirror is also provided at 45° in this tube to sight the bubble of bubble tube. Bubble tube is attached with vernier arm. When the line of sight is not horizontal the milled screw is operated till the bubble is bisected by the cross wire. Thus vernier moves from zero to some angle which is equal to the inclination of the line of sight.

A semi-circular graduated arc is fixed in position. The readings change from 0° to 60° (or 90°) in both directions. One direction gives the angle of elevation and the other angle of depression. This instrument can be used as hand level by setting the vernier to read zero on the graduated arc.

Then the screw is turned slowly so that the image of the right hand object coincides with the left hand object. Clamp the vernier. The reading on the vernier gives angle between two points directly.

If it is required to measure the vertical angle then the sextant is hold such that its arc lies in a vertical plane. Lower object is sighted directly and screw is turned until the image of higher object appears coinciding with the lower one.

Reference for Surveying Laboratory

1. Agor, R., A Text Book on Surveying and Levelling (in MKS units), Khanna Publishers, Delhi, 4th edition, 1987.
2. Clerk David, Plane and Geodetic Surveying for Engineers, Constable Press, London, 6th edition, 1969.
3. Davis, Reynold Earl, Surveying : Theory and Practice, McGraw Hill Book Co. Ltd., New York, 5th edition, 1966.
4. Kanetkar, T.P. and Kulkarni, S.V., Surveying and Levelling, Part I and II, United Book Corporation, Poona, 23rd revised and enlarged edition, 1975.
5. Punmia, B.C., Surveying : Part I and II, Standard Book Depot, Delhi, 6th edition, 1984.
6. Ripa, Louis Carl, Surveying Manual, McGraw Hill Publishing Co. Ltd., New York, 2nd edition, 1964.

SECTION 3

HYDRAULICS LABORATORY

Flow and fluid properties are studied in hydraulic laboratory. The scope and the importance of these experiments are as under.

Determination of energy and momentum coefficient helps in determining energy and momentum of flowing fluid. Without applying these coefficients a designer may reach to a wrong decision.

Actual discharge is determined by multiplying the theoretical discharge to a coefficient called discharge coefficient. This coefficient is determined in laboratory and it is different for different orifices, notches and weirs. Study of weirs, notches and orifice is helpful in designing of them in real life. Weirs are generally constructed on river bed to raise the water level. Notches are attached to canals to control the flow of water. Velocity distribution experiments gives the values of velocities at different points of a cross section. By means of velocity distribution the optimum depth of flow can be found out. Bernoulli's equation verification relates the area of cross section of flow and velocity of flow. So the diameter of pipes of water supply line or sewer line and the velocity of flow in them are regulated by Bernoulli's equation.

Hydraulic jump is the mean of dissipations of flow energy. If the velocity of fluid is very high, it may damage the bed and boundary. To prevent the bed and boundary being damaged, the velocity of flow is reduced by the hydraulic jump. There are many more applications of hydraulic jump.

Experiment No. 1

Object :

a) To determine the annular area between the rotameter tube and the float at different heights of the tube.

b) Measurement of volumetric flow rate using Rotameter.

Theory :

The rate of flow Q through rotameter is given by formula

$$Q = A \left[\frac{1}{C_d} 2g \frac{V_b}{A_b} \left(\frac{\rho_b}{\rho_f} - 1 \right) \right]^{\frac{1}{2}}$$

A is the annular area between the tube and the float at the reference point.

A_b = area of float at its maximum cross section

ρ_b, ρ_t = density of bob and fluid respectively

V_b = total volume of float

C_d = drag coefficient

Procedure : Part A

1. Known volume (V) of water is passed in to the tube and the corresponding hights of water (h) column measured.
2. Plot volume (V) vs height (h) of rotameter reading.
3. At any particular graduation find volume/height.
4. Measure the maximum cross sectional area of float (A).
5. Obtain (volume/height) — maximum cross-sectional area of float (A), i.e., annular area.

Part B

Rotameter reading versus volumetric flow rate.

1. Open the supply valve and allow the fluid to flow through rotameters.
2. Observe the position of float.
3. Collect the discharge in the bucket for a known time to calculate rate of flow.
4. Repeat your observations by adjusting the supply valve for increased flow for entire range of rotameter.
5. Calculate the values of C_d for different flow rates.
6. Plot rotameter reading versus volumetric flow rate.

Table of observations : Part A

Max. bob diameter_____

S. No.	Volume of water added	Total volume of water	Rotameter graduation reading (V)	Height of water column h

Calculations from the plot of V versus Height calculated.

S. No.	Rotameter graduation reading	Cross sectional area of tube	Annular area

Table of observations : Part B

Volume of float V_b _____

Density of float ρ_b _____

Density of fluid ρ_f _____

S. No.	Rotameter reading	Volume of water collected	Time of collection	Q	C_d

Results :

Questions :

1. What are the different forces that act on rotameter?
2. Can we use any other fluid in place of water? If yes, what are the changes that we have to make?

Experiment No. 2

Object :

To verify Stoke's law.

Apparatus/Equipments :

Calibrated glass cylinder (filled with glycerine), stop watch, balance, etc.

Theoretical background :

Stoke's law defines the rate of fall of a sphere through liquid. The velocity of a sphere falling freely in the liquid increases first under the action of gravity. This increase in the velocity results in to the viscous friction force which acts in the direction opposite to the motion of particle. So as the velocity increases, the frictional force also increases. Initially the magnitude of frictional force is negligible as compared to gravitational force but as particle travels in liquid its speed increases and so the frictional force increases. A stage is reached where the down ward force is equal to the upward force. Hence the net force on particle becomes zero. The velocity at this stage is called terminal velocity and it remains constant after the attainment of zero net force stage.

According to the Stoke's law the terminal velocity is given by

$$V = \frac{\gamma_s - \gamma_f}{18\,\mu} D^2$$

γ_s = specific wt. of sphere

γ_f = specific wt. of liquid

μ = viscosity of liquid

D = diameter of sphere.

Procedure :

1. Take 6 or 7 spheres and weigh them. Note down the room temperature also.
2. Measure the diameter of each sphere in three directions. Calculate the average diameter for each sphere.
3. Now release the sphere at the surface of liquid without any jerk, i.e., initial velocity of particle = 0.
4. Start the stop watch after the particle has travelled downward 15 to 20 cm in liquid column.
5. Note down the time taken and distance travelled by the particle.
6. Repeat the steps 3 to 5 for other particles (sphere) also.

Observations :

$\gamma_f =$ Temp. = $\mu =$

S. No.	Mass	Diameter			Distance travelled by the sphere	Time taken
		I	II	III		

Calculations :

S. No.	Diameter	Mass/Vol.	$\gamma_s = g \times$ density	$\gamma_f =$	V_{cal}	Distance/time $= V_{act}$

Results :

For a particle

  Actual velocity =

  Theoretical velocity =

Precautions :

1. The diameter of sphere should be measured in at least two directions.
2. The stop watch should be started after the particle has travelled some distance. If it is started before the attainment of terminal velocity, it might lead to wrong results.

Questions :

1. If initial velocity of particle, while releasing it at the surface of liquid is not zero, then what error would you encounter in the results and how would you overcome this situations?
2. For what value of Reynolds number, the Stokes law holds good?
3. What is Drag coefficient and how will you calculate it using Stoke's law?

Experiment No. 3

Object :

To verify Darcy's law.

Apparatus/Equipment :

Water supply mean, soil specimen (of which permeability is to be calculated), flow rate measuring tank, pressure measuring device, etc.

Theoretical background :

Any material containing continuously connected pores would permit the fluid to pass through itself. The property of material which permits fluid to percolate through is called its permeability. It is an important property of soil and its knowledge helps in the design of embankments and other hydraulic structures.

The Darcy's law states that the rate of flow Q, is proportional to the hydraulic gradient and the cross-sectional area.

$Q \propto iA$

$Q = k i A$ ...(1)

Q = flow rate

k = permeability

i = hydraulic gradient

A = cross-sectional area of soil specimen.

Hydraulic gradient, $i = \dfrac{\text{Head difference between two points}}{\text{Length of flow between two points}}$

$$i = \frac{h}{L} \qquad \qquad ...(2)$$

$$Q = \frac{V}{t} = \frac{\text{volume of water collected}}{\text{time of collection}}$$

$$= \frac{V}{t} = k \frac{h}{L} A$$

Therefore $k = \dfrac{VL}{thA}$ ...(3)

Procedure :

1. Put the soil sample in a container and compact it.
2. Pass the water in the upward direction and open the air valve so that the sample gets saturated and air bubbles are completely removed.
3. Close the air valve and let the water be flowing through for some time.
4. After the constant flow is established, collect water in measuring tank and observe the time collection.

5. Measure the head difference h between two points along the flow and also measure the distance between them.

6. Repeat the steps from 3 to 5 for different rate of water supply.

Observations :

1. Distance between the two points of which head difference is to be measured, L =
2. Cross sectional area of the soil sample, A =
3. Temperature of water =

Observation Table :

S. No.	Head difference	Discharge measurement	
		Vol. of water collected	Time of collection

Calculations :

1. Area of soil cross-section

2. Permeability $k = \dfrac{V}{t} \times \dfrac{L}{hA}$

Calculation Table :

S. No.	Permeability
1.	
2.	
3.	

Result :

Permeability of soil, k =

Precautions :

1. Each measurement should be taken after the establishment of constant flow.
2. There should be no entrapped air in manometer as well as in soil sample.

Experiment No. 4

Object :

To verify Bernoulli's equation.

Apparatus/Equipment :

Conduit of varying cross-sectional area fitted with peizometric tubes at regular intervals, water supply mean, flow rate measuring tank, etc.

Theoretical background :

For steady flow of an ideal fluid, the total energy head (i.e., the sum of geodetic, kinetic and pressure heads) is constant along a stream tube. According to Bernoulli,

total head $H = Z + \dfrac{P}{w} + \dfrac{V^2}{2g}$ is constant.

where Z = geodetic head

$\dfrac{P}{w}$ = pressure head

$\dfrac{V^2}{2g}$ = velocity head.

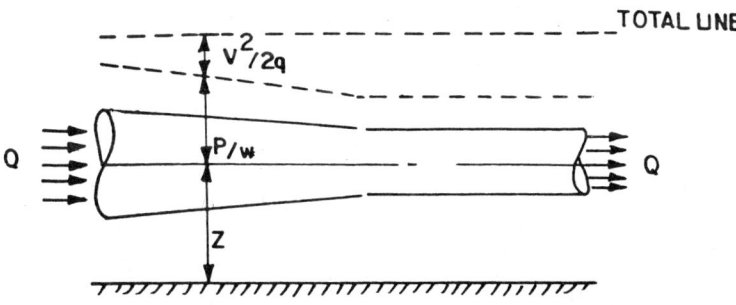

Procedure :

1. Note down the area of cross section of conduit at all peizometric points.
2. Open the supply valve and adjust the flow so that the water level in the inlet tank remains stable.
3. Measure the peizometric head for each peizometric points.
4. Collect the discharge for a known time and calculate the flow rate.
5. Repeat steps 2 to 4 for different discharges.
6. Plot hydraulic grade line and total energy line for each discharge.

Observations :

Area of measuring tank = length × width

= _____ × _____

S. No.	Rise in level of water in tank	Time of collection	Peizometric head at various sections								
			1	2	3	4	5	6	7	8	9
1											
2											
3											
Area of conduit at peizometric points											

Calculations :

1. Discharge (volume) of water = area of tank × rise in level.

2. Flow rate, $Q = \dfrac{\text{vol. of water}}{\text{time of collection}}$

3. Area of cross section at peizometric points =

4. Velocity of flow, $V = \dfrac{Q}{\text{area of peizometric pt.}}$

5. Velocity head = $\dfrac{V^2}{2g}$

6. Peizometric head = $\dfrac{P}{w} + Z$

7. Total head = (5) + (6) = $\dfrac{P}{w} + Z + \dfrac{V^2}{2g}$

S. No.	Discharge	Peizometric tube No. cross-sectional area	1	2	3	4	5	...	...
1.		Velocity Velocity head Peizometric head Total head							
2.									

Result :

The total head for a particular discharge is constant. Hence Bernoulli's theorem is proved.

Precautions :

1. There should be no entrapped air in Peizometric tubes.
2. There should be no leakage between upstream and downstream ends of the conduit.

Questions :

1. What are the assumptions made for verifying Bernoulli's theorem?
2. Can you derive Bernoulli's equation from general energy equation and Euler's equation of motion?
3. What happens to Bernoulli's equation, if
   (i) flow is steady but irrotational,
   (ii) flow is steady but rotational.

Experiment No. 5

Object :

To determine Darcy's friction factor 'f' of pipes of different diameters.

Apparatus/Equipment :

U-shaped glass tube filled partially with mercury, water supply mean, calibrated scale, etc.

Theoretical background :

When fluid flows through a conduit the frictional resistance offered to the flow depends on the roughness of the surface of conduit carrying the flow. In laminar flow, this frictional resistance is mostly due to viscous resistance of fluid. In turbulent flow it is due to resistance offered by viscosity of fluid and surface roughness of conduit.

The frictional resistance results into loss of head, h_f which is given by Darcy and Weisbach equation,

$$h_f = f\left(\frac{L}{D}\right)\frac{V^2}{2g} \qquad \qquad ...(1)$$

where

    f = Darcy's friction factor

    V = velocity of flow

    L = length of flow across which head loss is h_f

    D = diameter of pipe.

Head loss across the pressure tappings is measured by manometer having mercury as manometer fluid.

By applying simple pressure equation, pressure at C

$P_C = P_A + \rho_w g h_1 + \rho_{hg} g h_2 = P_B + \rho_w h_3 g$.

Pressure difference between A and B.

$-P_A + P_B = g\left[-\rho_w h_3 + \rho_w h_1 + \rho_{Hg} h_2\right]$

$P_B - P_A = g\left[\rho_{Hg} h_2 - \rho_w (h_3 - h_1)\right]$

$\qquad\quad = g\left[\rho_{Hg} h_2 - \rho_w h_2\right]$

$P_B - P_A = g h_2 \left[\rho_{Hg} - \rho_w\right] \qquad \qquad ...(2)$

This pressure difference $(P_B - P_A)$ is equivalent to height H_f on water column

$P_B - P_A = \rho_w H_f g = g h_2 (\rho_{Hg} - \rho_w)$

$H_f = (\rho_{Hg} - \rho_w) h_2 \qquad \qquad ...(3)$

where

    ρ_w = mass density of water

    ρ_{Hg} = mass density of manometer fluid.

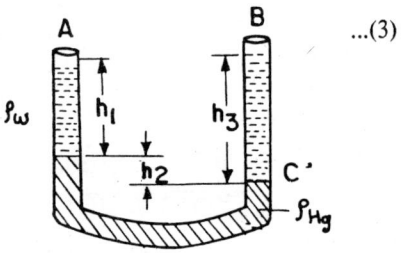

Procedure :

    1. Connect the manometer rubber tubes to pressure tappings.

2. Open the inlet valve by closing the outlet valve and remove entrapped air in manometer, if any.
3. Open the water supply and let the fluid flow through the pipe.
4. Let the flow stabilised, then collect the discharge for given time and observe the manometer reading.
5. Repeat the steps from 3 to 4 for six or seven different discharges.
6. Repeat steps (3) to (5) for other pipes.

Observations :

Diameter of pipe, D =
Length of pipe between pressure tappings, L =
Mass density of manometer fluid, ρ_{Hg} =
Mass density of water, ρ_w =

S. No.	Discharge collected	Time of collection	Manometer reading $h_2 = (h_3 - h_1)$
1.			
2.			
3.			
4.			

Calculations :

1. $H_f = \dfrac{(\rho_{Hg} - \rho_w)\, h_2}{\rho_w}$

2. Flow rate, $Q = \dfrac{\text{discharge collected}}{\text{time of collection}}$

3. Velocity of flow, $V = \dfrac{Q}{\text{area of conduit pipe}}$

4. $H_f \doteq f\left(\dfrac{L}{D}\right)\dfrac{V^2}{2g}$ or, $f = \dfrac{H_f\, D\, 2g}{L\, V^2}$

S. No.	h_2	H_f	V	$f = \dfrac{h_f\, D^2\, 2g}{L\, V^2}$
1.				
2.				
3.				

These observations are for one pipe only. Similar observations and calculations can be carried out for other pipes of different diameters and Darcy's friction factor 'f' can be calculated.

Result :

   Darcy's friction factor $f =$

Precautions :

   1. There should not be any entrapped air in apparatus while observing manometer reading.
   2. There should be no leakage anywhere in the pipe

Questions :

   1. What is 'hydraulic mean depth' or 'hydraulic radius'?
   2. Besides Darcy's method, what are the other formulae to calculate the friction factor 'f' for pipes due to roughness of pipe surfaces?
   3. Is the value 'f' constant for the pipes throughout? If not, then what factors does it depend on?

Experiment No. 6

Object :

To determine the coefficient of discharge, coefficient of velocity, coefficient of contraction and coefficient of resistance for an orifice under constant head.

Apparatus/Equipment :

Orifice fitted tank, volume measuring tank, hook gauge, etc.

Theoretical background :

An orifice is an opening made in side or bottom of fluid container and having the closed perimeter. Through the orifice the fluid may be discharged and it is used to measure the flow rate of fluid. The liquid approaching the orifice gradually converges towards it and emerges from it in the form of a jet. The cross sectional area of jet is less than that of the orifice since the motion of liquid particle close to the inner wall cannot change the direction abruptly at the orifice edge.

The section of jet at which the stream lines are straight, parallel to each other and having the minimum cross sectional area is known as Vena Contracta.

The ratio of area of jet at vena contracta and area of orifice is called the coefficient of contraction

$$C_c = \frac{A_c}{A} \qquad\qquad ...(1)$$

where

A_c = area of jet at vena contracta

A = area of orifice

Due to the friction the velocity of jet is reduced. So the actual velocity of the jet at vena contracta is less then that of the theoretical velocity. The ratio of the two is called the coefficient of velocity.

$$C_v = \frac{V}{V_{th}} \qquad\qquad ...(2)$$

$V_{th} = \sqrt{2gh}$

V_{th} = theoretical velocity

V = actual velocity

C_v = coefficient of velocity

Due to the effect of friction and due to the contraction of jet the actual discharge of liquid is less than the theoretical discharge. The ratio of them is called the coefficient of discharge.

$$C_d = \frac{Q}{Q_{th}}$$

$Q = A_c \times V$

$\qquad\qquad ...(3)$

$Q_{th} = A \times V_{th}$

$\qquad = A \times \sqrt{2gh}$

Q_{th} = theoretical discharge

Q = actual discharge

C_d = coefficient of discharge

Therefore

$$C_d = \left(\frac{A_c}{A}\right)\left(\frac{V}{V_{th}}\right) = \frac{Q}{A \times \sqrt{2gh}}$$

$$C_d = C_c \times C_v \qquad \qquad ...(4)$$

If x and y are the horizontal and vertical distances of a point from vena contracts respectively and V is the velocity of jet, g is the gravitational acceleration then the horizontal distance travelled by the liquid particle in time t will be

$$x = Vt \qquad \qquad ...(5)$$

and vertical distance y will be

$$y = \frac{gt^2}{2} \qquad \qquad ...(6)$$

From (5) and (6) $\quad x = V\sqrt{\dfrac{2y}{g}} \quad$ or, $\quad V = \sqrt{\dfrac{gx^2}{2y}}$

$$C_v = \frac{V}{V_{th}} = \frac{\sqrt{\dfrac{gx^2}{2y}}}{\sqrt{2gh}} = \sqrt{\frac{x^2}{4yh}} \qquad \qquad ...(7)$$

Procedure :

1. Open the supply valve in the orifice tank to attain the maximum depth of water.
2. Now allow the water to discharge through the orifice and adjust the supply valve in such a way that depth of water in tank remains constant.
3. When the depth in the tank stabilizes, collect the discharge in the measuring tank for a predetermined period of time. Read x and y, the co-ordinates of several points (at least 3) on jet.
4. Reduce slightly the discharge by supply valve and repeat step No. 3. Thus obtain readings for 4 to 5 different valve settings.
5. For each valve setting read the depth of water by peizometric tube.

Observations :

Diameter of orifice =   Area of measuring tank –

S. No.	Depth of water in orifice tank	Co-ordinates						Velocity				Rise in level of water in measuring tank	Time of collection
		x			y			V					
		I	II	III	I	II	III	I	II	III	mean		

Calculations :

$$V = \sqrt{\frac{x^2 g}{2y}}$$

$$V_{th} = \sqrt{2gh}$$

$$C_v = \frac{V}{V_{th}}$$

$$= \sqrt{\frac{x^2}{4yh}}$$

(a) Volume of water collected =

(b) Time taken in collecting water =

$$Q = \frac{(a)}{(b)}$$

$$C_d = \frac{Q}{Q_{th}}; \quad Q_{th} = A V_{th}; \quad C_c = \frac{C_d}{C_v}; \quad C_r = \frac{1}{C_v^2} - 1$$

Results :

Coefficient of discharge, C_d =

Coefficient of velocity, C_v =

Coefficient of contraction, C_c =

Coefficient of resistance, C_r =

Precautions :

1. There should not be any air bubble in the peizometric tube.
2. While taking the reading, the level of water in orifice tank must be constant.

Questions :

1. Define 'Vena Contracta'. Explain how it is developed.
2. What are the other methods for the determination of coefficient of velocity, C_v?

Experiment No. 7

Object :

To determine the coefficient of discharge of an orifice under varying head.

Apparatus/Equipment :

Water supply means, flow rate measuring tank, fluid container fitted with orifice at bottom, etc.

Theoretical background :

If the head over the orifice is not constant then flow becomes unsteady. As shown in figure, there is fluid in tank upto some height H_1. Let at any distance the liquid surface be at a height h above the orifice and let the liquid surface fall by a small amount dh in time dt. If A is the horizontal cross sectional area of the tank and Q is the flow rate, then

$$A \, dh = -Q \, dt \qquad \qquad \ldots(1)$$

If a = area of orifice, then

$$Q = C_d \, a \, \sqrt{2gh}$$

C_d = discharge coefficient

h = head over the orifice

$$A \, dh = -C_d \, a \, \sqrt{2gh} \, dt$$

$$dt = -\frac{A \, dh}{C_d \, a \, \sqrt{2gh}}$$

Time taken by liquid surface to fall from height H_1 to H_2

$$\int_0^t dt = -\frac{A}{C_d \, a \, \sqrt{2g}} \int_{H_1}^{H_2} \frac{1}{\sqrt{h}} \, dh$$

$$t = \frac{2A}{C_d \, a \, \sqrt{2g}} \left(-\sqrt{H_2} + \sqrt{H_1} \right) \qquad \qquad \ldots(2)$$

After H_2 the horizontal area of cross section tank changes linearly.

The cross-sectional area at height h_1 will be

$$= \left(B_2 + \frac{B_1 - B_2}{H_2} \times h_1 \right)^2$$

$$= \frac{[B_2 H_2 + (B_1 - B_2) \, h_1]^2}{H_2^2}$$

Time taken by liquid surface to fall from height H_2 to 0.

$$t = -\int_{H_2}^{0} \frac{A \, dh}{C_d \, a \, \sqrt{2gh}}$$

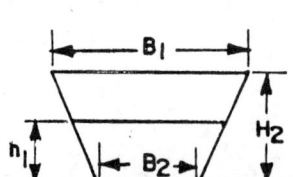

$$t = -\int_{H_2}^{0} \frac{\dfrac{[B_2H_2 + (B_1 - B_2)\,h]^2}{H_2^2}}{C_d\,a\,\sqrt{2gh}}\,dh$$

$$= -\frac{1}{a\,\sqrt{2g}\,C_d\,H_2^2}\int_{H_2}^{0} \frac{B_2^2\,H_2^2 + (B_1 - B_2)^2\,h^2 + 2B^2 H^2\,(B_1 - B_2)\,h\;dh}{\sqrt{h}}$$

$$= \frac{1}{a\,C_d\,(B_2H_2)^2\,\sqrt{2g}}\,2\,(B_2H_2)^2\,\sqrt{H_2} + \frac{2}{5}\,(B_1 - B_2)^2\,H_2^{5/2} + \frac{4}{3}\,B_2H_2\,(B_1 - B_2)\,H_2^{3/2}$$

$$= \frac{1}{a\,C_d\,\sqrt{2g}}\,2\,\sqrt{H_2}\,B_2^2 + \frac{2}{5}\,\frac{(B_1 - B_2)^2}{H_2^2}\,H_2^{5/2} + \frac{4}{3}\,\frac{(B_1 - B_2)\,B_2H_2}{H_2^2}\,H_2^{3/2}$$

If $K_1 = B_2$

$$K_2 = \frac{(B_1 - B_1)}{H_2}$$

$$t = \frac{1}{C_d\,\sqrt{2g}\,a}\,2K_1^2\,\sqrt{H_2} + \frac{2}{5}\,K_2^2\,H_2^{5/2} + \frac{4}{3}\,K_1K_2H_2^{3/2} \qquad \text{...(3)}$$

Total time taken from height H_1 to zero

$$t = (2) + (3)$$

$$= \frac{2A}{C_d\,a\,\sqrt{2g}}\,(\sqrt{H_1} - \sqrt{H_2}) + \frac{1}{C_d\,a\,\sqrt{2g}}\,2K_1^2\,\sqrt{H_2} + \frac{4}{3}\,K_1K_2H_2^{3/2} + \frac{2}{5}\,K_2^2H_2^{5/2} \qquad \text{...(4)}$$

where $A = B_1^2$.

Procedure :

1. Fill the water in the tank upto height H_1.
2. Release the valve of orifice and let the water discharge out of tank.
3. Collect the discharged water in the measuring tank.
4. Let the orifice tank be empty and note down the total emptying time (from height H_1).
5. Observe the emptying time of portion of tank for fixed cross sectional area and also of variable cross sectional area.

Observations :

Width of the tank, $B_1 =$

Area of tank, $A = B_1^2 =$

Dimension of tank at orifice, $B_2 =$

Initial head, $H_1 =$

Final head, $H_2 =$

Area of orifice, $a = B_2^2 =$

(a)	Emptying time of fixed cross-sectional area =
(b)	Emptying time of variable cross-sectional area =

Total emptying time = (a) + (b) =

Calculations :

For fixed cross-sectional area only

$$t_1 = \frac{2A}{C_d \, a \, \sqrt{2g}} (\sqrt{H_1} - \sqrt{H_2})$$

$$C_{d_1} = \frac{2A}{t_1 \, a \, \sqrt{2g}} (\sqrt{H_1} - \sqrt{H_2})$$

For variable cross-sectional area only

$$C_{d_2} = \frac{1}{t_2 \, \sqrt{2g} \, a} \, 2K_1^2 \sqrt{H_2} + \frac{2}{5} K_2^2 H_2^{5/2} + \frac{4}{3} K_1 K_2 H_2^{3/2}$$

For whole tank

Substitute the values in equation and determine C_{d_3} =

Result :

1. C_{d_1} =
2. C_{d_2} =
3. C_{d_3} =

Precautions :

1. Stop watch should be started as soon as the valve of orifice is opened.
2. There should be no leakage from anywhere for accurate measurement.

Experiment No. 8

Object :

To determine the coefficient of discharge 'C_d' of the V notch and to plot the calibration curve.

Apparatus/Equipment :

A rectangular channel at the end of which a V notch is fitted, water supply mean, flow rate measuring tank, hook gauge, etc.

Theoretical background :

A notch is the opening provided at the side or the bottom of the vessel. Notches are generally used to measure rate of flow of liquid from a tank or in a channel V notches are used to measure the low discharges.

From the figure,

$$\tan \theta/2 = \frac{x}{2\,(H-h)}$$

$$x = 2\,(H-h)\tan\theta/2 \qquad \qquad \text{...(i)}$$

The area of strip of dimensions x and dh is $= xdh$

Velocity of fluid flowing through the strip $= \sqrt{2gh}$

Discharge dQ through the strip

$$dQ = x\sqrt{2gh}\;dh$$

$$= [2\,(H-h)\tan\theta/2\sqrt{2gh}\;dh \qquad \qquad \text{...(ii)}$$

Actual discharge is less than the theoretical discharge. Therefore,

$$dQ_a = 2C_d\,(H-h)\tan(\theta/2)\sqrt{2gh}\;dh \qquad \qquad \text{...(iii)}$$

C_d = discharge coefficient

The total discharge Q_a over the V (triangular) notch

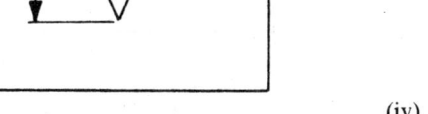

$$Q_a = \int_0^H 2\,(H-h)\tan\theta/2\,C_d\sqrt{2gh}\;dh$$

$$= 2\,C_d\sqrt{2g}\,\tan\theta/2\left[\frac{2}{3}Hh^{3/2} - \frac{2}{3}h^{5/2}\right]_0^H$$

$$= \frac{8}{15}C_d\sqrt{2g}\,\tan\theta/2\,H^{5/2} \qquad \qquad \text{...(iv)}$$

If the velocity of approach is to be taken into account then

$$Q_a = \frac{8}{15}C_d\sqrt{2g}\,\tan\theta/2\,[H_1^{5/2} - h_a^{5/2}] \qquad \qquad \text{...(v)}$$

$$H_1 = H + h_a$$

and $h_a = \dfrac{V_a^2}{2g}$, where V_a is velocity of approach.

Procedure :

1. Open the supply valve and close it immediately and let the water drain out upto the vertex of the notch. Observe the hook gauge reading. It is called zero reading, i.e., reading for zero flow.
2. Open the supply valve and wait till the head over the notch stabilizes. Now take the hook gauge reading and measure the flow rate.
3. Repeat the step (2) with different setting of valve to cover the entire range of head H.
4. Plot the calibration curve for V notch, i.e., curve between Q_a and H on log-log graph sheet. Determine the value of K and n.

$Q_a = KH^n$

$\log Q_a = \log K + n \log H$

This is the mathematical form of a straight line in cartesian coordinates, $Y = C + mX$

Hence by taking $\log Q_a$ as dependent variable and height as independent variable, plot

$\log Q_a = f(\log H)$ so that

K = antilog of the Y-intercept

n = slope of the line.

Also plot H vs. C_d.

Observations :

1. Angle of notch θ =
2. Initial hook gauge reading =
3. Dimensions of the measuring tank

      Length =   Width =

S. No.	Final hook gauge reading	Measuring tank reading		Time of collection
		Initial reading	Final reading	
1.				
2.				
3.				
4.				
5.				

Calculations :

1. Head over the notch = Final – Initial hook gauge reading.

2. Actual discharge = $\dfrac{\text{Area of measuring tank} \times \text{rise of water}}{\text{time of collection}}$

3. Theoretical discharge = $\dfrac{8}{15} C_d \sqrt{2g} \tan \theta/2 \, H^{5/2}$

4. Coefficient of discharge $C_d = \dfrac{\text{Actual discharge}}{\text{Theoretical discharge}}$

Table of calculations :

S. No.	Head over the notch	Actual discharge	Q_{th}	C_d
1.				
2.				
3.				

Result :

The range of C_d =

K =

n =

Precautions :

1. Zero readings should be taken when there is no flow over the notch.
2. For the accurate measurement of discharge there should be no leakage at any valve.
3. Apparatus should be levelled.

Questions :

1. What is a notch? How are the notches classified?
2. Define velocity of approach. How can you account for it while computing the discharge over the V notch?
3. What are the advantages of using V-notch over rectangular notch.
4. What happens, if
   (i) approach velocity is not taken into consideration,
   (ii) rectangular notch is used instead of V-notch for measuring the discharge?

Experiment No. 9

Object :

To determine the coefficient of discharge of the broad crested weir.

Apparatus/Equipment :

Water supply mean, open channel with broad crested weir, flow measuring device, i.e., rectangular notch, etc.

Theoretical background :

A weir having a wide crest (B > 0.5H) is known as broad crested weir. Generally the weirs are used to measure the flow rate and to raise the level of water of rivers on upstream side.

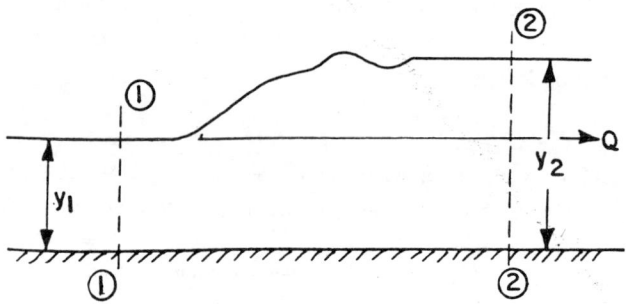

As the water flows over a broad crested weir the water surface drops from H on the upstream of the weir to h over the crest of weir. Since the cross sectional area of flow reduces at the weir therefore the velocity at the weir increases. Let the velocity of flow at weir is V neglecting the approaching velocity of flow and applying the Bernoulli's equation at section 1-1 and 2-2.

$$H = h + V^2/2g$$
$$V = \sqrt{2g\,(H-h)} \qquad \qquad ...(1)$$

If L is the length of the crest of the weir then discharge over the broad crested weir is

$$Q_{th} = Q = Lh\,\sqrt{2g\,(H-h)} \qquad \qquad ...(2)$$

But the actual discharge over the broad crested weir is less than that of given by equation (2).

$$Q_{act} = C_d\,Lh\,\sqrt{2g\,(H-h)} \qquad \qquad ...(3)$$

where C_d is the coefficient of discharge.

The flow adjusts itself to have maximum discharge for the available head H. Therefore the condition for maximum discharge Q for a constant head H may be obtained by differentiating the equation (3) with respect to h and equating $\dfrac{dQ}{dh}$ to zero.

$$\frac{dQ}{dh} = C_d\,L\,\sqrt{2g}\left[\sqrt{(H-h)} - \frac{1}{2}\,h\,(H-h)^{\frac{1}{2}}\right] = 0$$

$$\sqrt{(H-h)} = \frac{h}{2\sqrt{(H-h)}} \quad \text{or,} \quad 2(H-h) = h$$

$$h = \frac{2}{3}H \qquad \qquad \qquad ...(4)$$

Introducing the values of h in equation (3) we get

$$Q_{act} = 1.70\, C_d\, \frac{3}{2}\, LH^{3/2} \qquad \qquad ...(5)$$

If velocity of approach V_a is considered then equation (5) may be modified as

$$Q = 1.70\, C_d\, L\, H_1^{3/2}$$

where $H_1 = H + h_a = H + \dfrac{V_a^2}{2g}$.

Procedure :

1. Keep the tail gate of the channel open and ensure the non submergence of weir.
2. Open the supply valve and let the water level equal to the crest of rectangular notch. Take the initial hook gauge reading.
3. Open the supply valve and when the flow stabilizes, locate a point on upstream of the weir which is free to the effect of draw down. All readings for H must be taken at this point. Similarly locate a point for h along the crest of weir.
4. Read h and H for the weir and also obtain the head over the calibrated rectangular notch.
5. Change the valve setting and repeat step 4. Obtain the sets of observations for 5 to 7 different settings of supply valve.
6. Plot the calibration curve for weir on log-log paper.
7. Compare the h with the critical depth 'h_c'.

Observations :

Width of the weir, B =
Length of the weir, L =
Height of the weir, Z =
Pointer gauge reading for the crest of the weir =
Initial hook gauge reading for the rectangular notch =

S. No.	Final hook gauge reading	Final pointer gauge reading	
		Upstream	Over the crestor
1.			
2.			
3.			

Calculations :

Head over the calibrated notch :

From the calibration curve discharge

$Q_a =$

H = Final pointer gauge reading on upstream – initial pointer gauge reading (at bed).

h = Final pointer gauge reading at weir – initial pointer gauge reading.

Theoretical discharge :

$Q_{th} = 1.70 \, L \, H^{3/2}$

Coefficient of discharge, $C_d = \dfrac{Q_a}{Q_{th}}$

Critical depth corresponding to Q_a

$h_c = \left(\dfrac{Q_a^2}{L^2 g}\right)^{1/3}$ (derived from eqn. 2 and 4 and replacing Q by Q_a)

Calculations :

S. No.	Head over the notch	Q_a	H	h	Q_{th}	C_d	h_c for given Q_a
1.							
2.							
3.							
4.							

Result :

$C_d =$

Precautions :

1. Hook gauge and pointer gauge reading should be measured accurately.
2. Before making the observations for Q and h, it should be confirmed that stream lines are parallel to the top of the broad crested weir.

Experiment No. 10

Object :

To study the formation of hydraulic jump.

Apparatus/Equipment :

Water supply, flow rate measuring device, transparent channel with sluice gate at inlet and outlet.

Theoretical background :

Hydraulic jump is a sudden and turbulent passage of water from a super critical state to a sub critical state. It is useful mean to dissipate the energy of flowing water which other wise may cause damage to bed on which water is flowing. Since the unknown amount of energy dissipates, energy equation cannot be used to analyse the hydraulic jump and hence momentum equation is used in analysis of it.

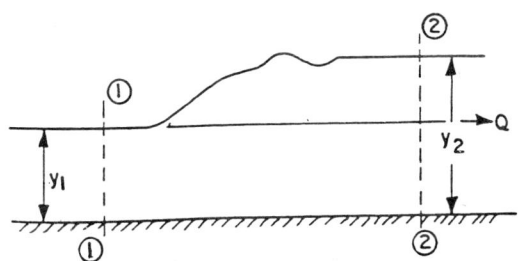

Applying the momentum equation between 1-1 and 2-2

$$\rho \, g \, A_2 \, Z_2 - \rho \, g \, A_1 \, Z_1 = \rho \, Q \, (V_1 - V_2)$$

$$\frac{Q^2}{g \, A_1} + A_1 \, Z_1 = \frac{Q^2}{g \, A_2} + A_2 \, Z_2$$

$$F_1 = F_2 \qquad \qquad ...(1)$$

F_1 and F_2 are specific force at section 1-1 and 2-2. For the rectangular channel

$$A_1 = B \, Y_1; \quad A_2 = B \, Y_2$$

$$Z_1 = \frac{Y_1}{2}; \quad Z_2 = \frac{Y_2}{2}$$

$$\frac{Q^2}{g \, (B \, Y_1)} + \frac{B \, Y_1^2}{2} = \frac{Q^2}{g \, (B \, Y_2)} + B \, Y_2^2 \qquad \qquad ...(2)$$

$$\frac{Q}{B} = q$$

$$\frac{2 \, q^2}{g} = Y_1 \, Y_2 \, (Y_1 + Y_2) \qquad \qquad ...(3)$$

Equation (3) can be written as

$$\frac{Y_2}{Y_1} = \frac{1}{2}\left[-1 + \sqrt{\frac{8\,q^2}{g\,Y_1^3}}\,\right]$$

Froude number before the hydraulic jump $= \dfrac{q}{g\,Y_1^3} = F_r$

Therefore $\dfrac{Y_2}{Y_1} = \dfrac{1}{2}\left[-1 + \sqrt{x + 8F_r^2}\,\right]$ ...(4)

The loss of energy between 1-1 and 2-2

$$\Delta E = Y_1 + \frac{V_1^2}{2g} - \left(Y_2 + \frac{v_2^2}{2g}\right)$$

$$= \left[Y_1 + \frac{Q^2}{2g\,(B\,Y_1)^2} - Y_2 - \frac{Q^2}{2g\,(B\,Y_2)^2}\right]$$

$$\Delta E = \frac{Q^2}{2g}\frac{(Y_2^2 - Y_1^2)}{(Y_1\,Y_2)^2} - (Y_2 - Y_1)$$

From equation (3) $\dfrac{q^2}{2g} = \dfrac{Y_1\,Y_2\,(Y_1 + Y_2)}{4}$

$$\Delta E = \frac{(Y_1 + Y_2)\,(Y_2^2 - Y_1^2)}{4\,Y_1 Y_2} - (Y_2 - Y_1)$$

$$= \frac{(Y_2 - Y_1)}{Y_1\,Y_2}\,(Y_1^2 + Y_2^2 + 2\,Y_1 Y_2) - 4\,Y_1 Y_2$$

$$\Delta E = \frac{(Y_2 - Y_1)^3}{Y_1\,Y_2}$$ ...(5)

Procedure :

1. Adjust supply valve, sluice gate for inlet and outlet so that there forms a stable hydraulic jump in the flume.
2. Take the pointer gauge reading for the bottom of the channel and water surface elevation at pre-jump section and post jump section.
3. Measure the length of jump i.e. distance between section 1-1 and 2-2.
4. Measure the discharge by collecting the water in a tank of known cross sectional area for known period of time.
5. Repeat the step 1 to 4 for other positions of valve and gates. Take about 8 sets of observations.

Observations :

1. Width of the channel =
2. Hook gauge reading for the bottom of the channel =
3. Cross-sectional area of water collecting tank =

S. No.	Hook gauge reading		Height of water in tank	Time of collection	Length of jump
	Pre-jump	Post-jump			
1.					
2.					
3.					

Calculations :

S. No.	Y_1	Y_2	Q	$q = Q/B$	Y_2/Y_1	$F_r = q \sqrt{g\, Y_1}$	$\Delta E = \dfrac{(Y_2 - Y_1)^3}{Y_1\, Y_2}$
1.							
2.							
3.							

Result :

Froude No., F_r =

Energy loss =

Precautions :

1. Jump should be a stable jump.
2. Length and height of jump must be measured accurately.
3. Plot the graph between $\dfrac{Y_2}{Y_1}$ and F_r on ordinary graph paper and on the same graph paper plot the line represented by equation (4).

Questions :

1. What are the different applications of hydraulic jump?
2. Why we can't apply the conservation of energy?

Experiment No. 11

Object :

To study the losses in head h_l and to obtain the factor f for the following cases :

    a) friction of pipe wall,

    b) gradual expansion or contraction of cross-section of pipe,

    c) sudden expansion and contraction of cross-section of pipe,

    d) losses in bends.

Apparatus/Equipment

83 meter pipe line, venturimeter, peizometric switch board, manometer board with 17 pressure tappings, etc.

Theoretical background :

Taking energy losses h_l into account the Bernoulli's equation for steady flow is

$$p_1 + z_1 + \frac{v_1^2}{2g} = p_2 + z_2 + \frac{v_2^2}{2g} + h_l$$

Hence, the loss of head

$$h_l = p_1 - p_2 + v_1^2 - \frac{v_2^2}{2g} + z_1 - z_2$$

The head loss h_l is found to depend on the pipe properties and is proportional to the expression $\dfrac{v^2}{2g}$ such as in the cases mentioned below :

Case A : Friction in straight pipe of constant diameter :

$$h_l = f\frac{l}{d} \cdot \frac{v^2}{2g}$$

where

    l = length of pipe

    d = diameter of the pipe

    f = friction factor

    Hence, the friction factor

$$f = \frac{2g}{v^2} \cdot \frac{d}{l} h_l$$

Case B : Gradual expansion or contraction :

According to the expression for h_l for an elementary length of dx as per case A, the head loss is

$$dh_l = f\frac{dx}{d} \frac{v^2}{2g}$$

With $d = dx = d_2 x + d_1 \dfrac{1-x}{1}$ and $v = v(x) = \dfrac{4Q}{\pi} \dfrac{d^2}{x}$ the integration for $x = 0$ to $x = 1$ gives

$$h_l = \frac{f l \dfrac{d_2^2}{l} d_1^2 \dfrac{d_2 + d_1}{v^2}}{4 \dfrac{d_1^2}{2g}}$$

Hence, the friction factor

$$f = 2g \frac{4 d_1^2 h_1}{v^2} 1 d_2^2 + d_1^2 d_2 + d_1$$

Case C : Sudden expansion or contraction :

By means of momentum equations, h_l follows as

$$h_l = f v_1 - v_2 \, 2g$$

$$h_l = f \left(\frac{d_2}{d_1}\right)^2 \frac{v_2^2}{2g}$$

where f is depending not only on the friction properties of the boundaries but also on the ratio $\dfrac{d_2}{d_1}$.

The friction factor is then :

$$f = 2g \, h_l \, \frac{d_2}{d_1} - 1 \, v_2^2$$

Case D : Bends :

Here again the loss can be described in terms of

$$h_l = f \frac{v^2}{2g}$$

where $f = f(R, d)$ depends on the friction properties as well as on the parameters R and d.

The friction factor, therefore, is

$$f = 2g \frac{h_l}{v^2}$$

The experimental set-up :

The experimental set-up consists of an 83 meter pipe line, a venturimeter, a peizometric switch board, and a manometer board with scale. The line consists of 4 inch and 8 inch diameter pipes and includes attachments for gradual expansion and contraction, sudden expansion and contraction, vertical and horizontal bends. 17 pressure tappings are connected via the switch board to a manometer board with scale and air relief valves. Between sections 18 and 19 a venturimeter is installed. The pressure tappings of the section A and B refer respectively to the pressure at entrance and throat of the venturimeter. The referring pressure difference at the U-pipe 'AB' of the manometer board is used for calculation of the discharge. The flow is regulated by the two valves 1 and 2 and controlled by two pressure gauges 1 and 2 attached near to the valves.

Procedure :

1. Open valve 1 completely.
2. Ascertain that the system is free of air bubbles. For that purpose open the air relief valves on top of

the manometer pipes and switch the pointers of the selector successively from one tapping to the other.

3. Open valve 2. Ascertain that there is a small pressure left at pressure gauge 2. Close the air relief valve slowly.

4. Take the readings h_a and h_b at the U pipe "AB" of the manometer board.

5. Switch the pointer of the switch board upon 1 and take the readings h_1 and h_2 of section 1 at the U-pipe 1 of the manometer board.

6. Switch the adjuster upon 4 and the readings h_1 and h_2 for section 4, and continue in this way upto the readings for section 35. Note that for the readings 17 to 30 the readings have to be taken from the U-pipe 2, and for the section 35 from U-pipe 3.

7. Close at first valve 2 and thereafter valve 1.

Observations :

1. Diameter of the smaller pipe =
2. Diameter of the larger pipe =
3. Manometer reading at A =
4. Manometer reading at B =
5. Specific weight of the liquid =
6. Specific weight of the water =

S. No.	D	Z	$\dfrac{v^2}{2g}$	h_1	h_2	δh	$\Sigma\,\delta h$	H

(Same set of observations is to be recorded for 35 sections)

Calculations :

a) Discharge :

The readings $(h_a - h_b)$ at the manometer pipe 'AB' represents the difference of pressure at the venturimeter in height of mercury column. Multiplying with the difference of the specific weights of mercury and water, we get the pressure drop

$$P_a - P_b = (h_a - h_b)\,(\gamma_m - \gamma_w)$$

Thus, with the known values of $C_v = 0.965$ (as per DIN 1952), d, D, g, and $\gamma_w = 1$, the discharge will be

$$Q = 4585\,\sqrt{h_a - h_b}$$

b) Head losses :

In each of the 17 measuring sections the energy head H related to the datum line can be calculated.

$$v = \frac{Q}{A} = Q\,\frac{4}{\pi\,d^2}$$

$$p = z_0 + h_1 - z\,\gamma_w + \delta h\,\gamma_m$$

$$\gamma_w = 1$$

$$\gamma_m = 13.6$$

$$H = v^2\,2g + z - z_0 + \frac{p}{\gamma_w}$$

$$= v^2\,2g + h_1 + \partial h + \frac{\gamma_m}{\gamma_w}$$

The head loss in between two measuring sections with the sequence numbers m and n thus becomes

$$h_l = \partial h = H_m - H_n$$

If in between m and n there is no further section marked in the set-up, that is, if $n = m + 1$, the friction factor f can be calculated straightaway according to the respective formula given above.

However, if there are in between the sections m and n other sections marked, that means the friction conditions are non-uniform in the reach concerned, the total head loss has to be subdivided before calculation of the different friction factors.

c) Calculation of friction factor f :

The expression for the friction factor f can be given the general form

$$f = K\,\frac{h_l}{l}$$

where the definition of K depends on type of loss as follows :

Case A : Straight pipe of diameter d

$$K = \frac{d}{\left(\dfrac{v^2}{2g}\right)}$$

Case B : Gradual expansion or contraction of a pipe from diameter d_1 to d_2 ($d_2 > d_1$)

$$K = 4\,\frac{d_1^2}{d_2^2 + d_1^2}\,d_2 + d_1\,\frac{v^2}{2g}$$

Case C: Sudden expansion or contraction of a pipe from diameter d_1 to d_2 ($d_2 > d_1$) and ($l = 1$)

$$K = \frac{1}{\left(\dfrac{d_2}{d_1}\right)^2 - 1}\,\frac{v^2}{2g}$$

Case D : Bends of a pipe of diameter d

$$K = \frac{1}{\left(\dfrac{v^2}{2g}\right)}$$

S. No.	δH	h_l	K	l	$f = h_l \dfrac{K}{l}$

(Similarly do the calculation for all the 35 sections)

Results :

Energy loss (friction factor) due to friction of pipe wall =

Energy loss due to sudden change in cross-sectional area =

Energy loss due to gradual change in cross-sectional area =

Energy loss due to bends =

Total energy loss =

Experiment No. 12

Object :

To calculate the coefficient of velocity and momentum for a steady turbulent open channel flow and to obtain the velocity profile at a given section of flow.

Apparatus/Equipment :

Water supply mean, flow measuring tank, pointer gauges and current meter, etc.

Theoretical background :

The velocity profile over the flow section of a viscous fluid in motion is non-uniform due to the non-slip condition at the boundaries.

The shape of $v(y)$ depends on many factors, e.g., geometry and roughness of boundaries.

The average velocity

$$v = v \frac{dA}{A} = \frac{Q}{A}$$

is a very doubtful reference value for more exact computations. Therefore, in the case of velocity head and momentum certain correction factors are introduced :

Velocity head, $h_v = \dfrac{v^2}{2g}$

Momentum, $J = \dfrac{v^2}{A}$

The factors α = coefficient of velocity distribution and β = coefficient of momentum distribution can be determined if the point velocities are known.

Coefficient of velocity distribution

$$h_v = \frac{v^2}{2g}$$

is the velocity head for a horizontal stream tube of section dA according to Bernoulli's equation. Multiplication with $d_w = v\, dA\, \gamma_m$ gives the kinetic energy passing dA per unit time

$$h_v\, v\, dA = v^3\, dA\, \frac{\gamma_m}{2g}$$

Integrating over the total area

$$h_v\, v\, dA = v^3\, \frac{dA}{2g}$$

gives the velocity head $h_v = \alpha \dfrac{v^2}{2g}$

And, hence, the coefficient of velocity distribution

$$\alpha = \frac{\sum v^3\, \delta A}{v^3\, A}$$

Coefficient of momentum distribution :

Equating the correct term for the total momentum with the corrected one

$$\rho \, v \, dQ = \rho \, v \, Q$$

gives the coefficient of momentum distribution

$$\beta = \frac{\sum v^2 A}{v^2 A}$$

Procedure :

1. Take the zero reading H_{a_o}, H_{c_o} of the point gauges. Measure the width w of the flume and fix the current meter to the point gauge.
2. Allow a certain discharge to flow.
3. Take the readings H_{c_1} and H_{b_1} and calculate the flow depth $h = h_{b_1} - h_{b_0}$.
4. Calculate the coordinates of the measuring points X_i, Y_i and enter into table.
5. Set current meter at point 11 for a time T
6. Put automatic counter into operation and note down the number of revolutions n. Use stop watch.
7. Continue the procedure (steps 5 to 6) for the other measuring points.

Observations :

Initial head of water at a = H_{a_0} =

Initial head at b = H_{b_0} =

Initial head at c = H_{c_0} =

Final head at a = h_{a_1} =

Final head at b = H_{b_1} =

Final head at c = H_{c_1} =

Width of the tank = w =

Area of the section = A/15

Attachments :

Propeller No.	Diameter D	Revolutions n	Velocity v
1.	50	< 5.33 > 5.33	0.0565 * n + 0.035 0.0550 * n + 0.043
2.	50	< 1.08 > 1.08	0.0943 * n + 0.030 0.1026 * n + 0.021
3.	50	< 0.56 0.56 > n > 2.50 > 2.50	0.2197 * n + 0.030 0.2498 * n + 0.013 0.2530 * n + 0.005

Calculations :

Water depth $h = H_{b_0} - H_{b_1}$

Area $A = h\,w\,10000$

del area $= A/15$

Weir head $h_w = H_{c_0} - H_{c_1}$

Discharge $Q = f h_w$ from calibration chart

Average velocity, $v = \dfrac{Q}{A}$ regarded as the corrected value.

Point velocities for $n = \dfrac{N}{T}$

$v_m = f(n)$ from the calibration chart of the current meter of the corresponding equation

Average velocity $v_m = \delta A \sum \dfrac{v_m}{A}$

Measuring error $e = \dfrac{(v - v_m)\,100}{v}$

Correction factor $C_v = \dfrac{v}{v_m}$

Corrected velocity $v = c_v\,v_m$

Velocity distribution coefficient, $\alpha = \dfrac{\sum v^3\,dA}{v^3\,A}$

Momentum distribution coefficient, $\beta = \dfrac{\sum v^2\,dA}{v^2\,A}$

N for T = 50 secs	Y_1	− 16.0	− 8.0	0.00	8.00	16.0

(Similarly make the calculation table for $n = N/T$, $V_{measured}$, $V_{corrected} = C_v V_{measured}$, V^2 and V^3).

Result :

Velocity distribution coefficient, $\alpha =$

Momentum distribution coefficient, $\beta =$

Experiment No. 13

Object :

To determine the coefficient of permeability K and the pressure potential for a rectangular prismatic aquifer with a circular well in its centre. Further to show, how far Dupuit's equation for steady radial flow through an unconfined aquifer into a well is applicable.

Apparatus/Equipment :

Two masonry supply tanks linked with a flume filled with sieved sand, pressure gauges, etc.

Theoretical background:

Dupuit's equation for steady radial flow can be derived from Darcy's equation under the assumption that the vertical velocity component w is neglected.

Dupuit's equation $Q = \pi K h^2 - h_o^2 r - r_o$

For steady conditions, Q = constant is known from a discharge measurement of the well. Then the coefficient of permeability K can be calculated if the water table in the discharge r_0 and r from the centre of the well is known.

$$K = Q \ln \frac{\dfrac{r}{r_o}}{\pi h_2 - h_o^2}$$

K is constant for a given Q. Dupuit's equation describes the shape of the water table.

$$h = h(r) = \sqrt{Q \ln \frac{r/r_0}{\pi K + h_o^2}}$$

The inverse of this function furnishes for h = constant, equipotential lines

$$r = r(h) \, r_o \exp \left(K \pi \frac{h^2 - h_o^2}{Q} \right)$$

In the present experiment the ground water table and the discharge is measured :

$h = h(X, Y); \quad Q$ = constant

The permeability K is found from equation (2). The contour lines of the surface $h(X, Y)$ are to be compared with the corresponding circles as per equation (4).

Procedure :

1. Open valves 2, 3, 4 and 5 completely.
2. Open valve 1 and adjust until levels in the tanks (peizometers 1 to 89) are equal and constant.
3. Ascertain that all peizometric connections are entirely filled with water. Use section pump for removal of entrapped air.
4. Open syphon valve 6 and wait until the entire sand is fully saturated. This condition is fulfilled when the water level in the well remains constant.

5. Measure discharge Q by collecting a volume V_1 of water for known time t_1 in a container. Repeat this twice and enter values V_i and t_i in a container. Repeat this twice and enter values V_i and t_i ($i = 1, 2, 3$).

6. Note down the peizometric reading h_i of the manometer boards (points $i = 1$ to 89)

Observations :

Bottom level of well, $H_{w_0} =$

Water level of well, $H_w =$

Peizometer head at the point $i = 1, 2, 3$ 89

Measured outflow volume, V_i (for $i = 1, 2, 3$) =

Corresponding time interval, $t_i =$

Radius of the well, $r_0 =$

Calculations :

Discharge, $Q = \dfrac{2V_i}{t_i}$ for $i = 1...3$

Water depth of the well, $h_0 = H_w - H_{w_0}$

Permeability K can be calculated with the peizometer readings h_1 of the points $i = 26, 28, 33, 34, 50, 60, 62$.

From equation (2)

$$K = Q \ln \frac{\dfrac{r}{r_0}}{\pi\, h^2 - h_o^2} = Q\, 2.303 \log \frac{r}{r_0} \pi\, h^2 - h_o^2$$

where H is assumed as the average of H and

$r = \sqrt{X^2 - Y^2}$ = Constant

Equipotential lines : For the Dupuit's case of radial flow computed from equation (1)

$$\log \frac{r}{r_0} = \frac{\pi\, K\, (h^2 - h_o^2)}{2.302\, Q}$$

$$= C_1\, (h^2 - h_o^2)$$

with $C_1 = \dfrac{K}{Q\, 2.302}$

Calculation table for discharge Q :

Description	1	2	3
V_i			
t_i			
$Q_i = \dfrac{V_i}{t_i}$			
$Q = \dfrac{2}{3} Q_i$			

Calculation table for permeability K :

Points i	26	28	33	34	50	60	62
X_i							
Y_i							
$r_i = \sqrt{X_i^2 + Y_i^2}$							
$\log r_i$							
$\log r_i - \log r_o$							
H_i							
H_i^2							
$H_i^2 - H_o^2$							
$K = A \dfrac{\log \dfrac{r_i}{r_o}}{H_i^2 - H_o^2}$							

Calculation table for the equipotential lines according to Dupuit :

h	h^2	$\log \dfrac{r}{r_o}$	$\dfrac{r}{r_o}$	r
30				
32				
34				
36				
38				
40				
42				
44				
46				
48				
50				

Result :

Average value of permeability, K (average) =

Experiment No. 14

Object :

To determine different Raynolds numbers in the range where the laminar flow conditions change over to the turbulent flow condition.

Apparatus/Equipment :

A glass tube of diameter d, supply tank with bell mouth entrance, injection tank, flow collecting tank, etc.

Theoretical background :

The results of different scaled hydraulic models can only be compared if the corresponding flow conditions are dynamically similar. This is under the condition that the corresponding linear dimensions are geometrically similar, i.e., $l_a = \gamma\, l_b$

The forces under consideration are :
1. Inertia forces
2. Gravity forces
3. Friction forces
4. Capillary forces

Flow in closed circular conduits, gravity and capillary forces can be neglected without having any changes. The inertia and the friction forces then to be taken into account can be written in the form :

where d_m = mass element

a = acceleration

ρ = mass density

l = any characteristic length

t = time period

dF = elemental area

μ = molecular viscosity

ν = kinematic viscosity

These forces have to bear a constant ratio for the considered flow

$Fi\,(a)/Fi\,(b) = Ff\,(a)/Ff\,(b)$

i.e., inertia force is equal to the friction force.

With $v = \dfrac{l}{t}$ it becomes

$$\frac{l_a\, v_a}{\nu\, a} = \frac{l_b\, v_b}{\nu\, b}$$

Hence, a constant for both cases (Reynolds No.)

$$R_e = \frac{l\, v}{\nu}$$

In other words, two geometrical flow systems subject only to friction and inertia forces are dynamically similar if both have the same Reynolds number.

Since R_e is a characteristic value for the type of flow, it can also be used for the numerical description of some outstanding flow patterns which have been described earlier physically as laminar and turbulent.

For pipe flow, the following was found by experiment :

R_e < 2000 laminar flow

R_e = 2380 lower critical number

2000 < R_e < 4000 critical zone

R_e = 4000 upper critical number

4000 < R_e < 5000 transition zone

R_e < 5000 turbulent flow.

The decision whether laminar, transition or turbulent flow takes place can be made by observation of a fine stream of dye injected into a steady pipe flow :

Laminar — the dye stream moves as straight line

Transition — the dye stream wavers

Turbulent — the dye stream diffuses throughout the tube.

Procedure :

1. Open valves 1 and 2, and allow water to flow into the supply tank, and adjust by valve 2 to maintain constant head. Close valve 4.
2. Open the gate valve 5 gently a little to allow a very small discharge into the glass tube.
3. Pour dye into the container and open gently valve 3 a little.
4. Wait until the movement of the dye jet has reached equilibrium.
5. Take 2 readings h_1, h_2 at the manometer tube of the collecting tank within a measured time interval δt ($\geq$ 30).
6. Observe the flow condition in the tube, i.e., whether laminar or turbulent and make a note of it.

Calculations :

With the readings h_1, h_2, δt, the known diameter D of the pipe and the area A of the collecting tank, the Reynolds number can be calculated as follows :

Discharge $Q = \dfrac{h_2 - h_1}{\delta t \, At}$

Velocity $v = \dfrac{Q}{A}$

R_e number $= \dfrac{v \, D}{v}$ with v = 0.0101

Calculation table :

Run No.	1	2	3	4	5
h_1					
h_2					
δt					
$h_2 - h_1$					
$Q = \dfrac{h_2 - h_1}{t\,At}$					
$v = \dfrac{Q}{A}$					
$R_e = \dfrac{v\,D}{v}$					
Remark					

Result :

Flow in run 1 =
Flow in run 2 =
Flow in run 3 =
Flow in run 4 =
Flow in run 5 =

Reference for Hydraulics Engineering Laboratory

1. Arora K.R., Hydraulic and Fluid Mechanics and Hydraulic Machines, Standard Book Depot, Delhi, 3rd edition, 1980.
2. Barna P.S., Fluid Mechanics for Engineers, Planum Press, New York, 3rd edition, 1969.
3. Brater E.F. and King H.W., Handbook of Hydraulic, McGraw Hill Book Co. Ltd., New York, 6th edition, 1976.
4. Chow, Ven. Tc, Open Channel Hydraulics, McGraw Hill Book Co. Ltd., Tokyo, Kogakusha, 4th edition, 1967.
5. Dave R.M., Hydraulics and Introduction to Fluid Mechanics, Acharya Press, Baroda, 2nd edition, 1965.
6. Madani T.B., Practical Hydraulics and its Applications, Grindlays Bank, Bombay, 1949.
7. Modi, P.N. and Seth, S.M., Hydraulics and Fluid Mechanics including Hydraulic Machines, Standard Book Depot, Delhi, 24th revised and enlarged edition, 1986.
8. Rohde, F.G., Hydraulic Engineering Laboratory Experiment Manual, part I and II, Indian Institute of Technology, Madras. Deptt of Civil Engineering, 1st edition, 1976.
9. Likhi S.K., Hydraulic Laboratory Manual, Tata McGraw Hill Publishing Co. Ltd., New Delhi, 3rd edition, 1982.

Experiment No. 15

Object

1. To study the boundary layer velocity profile.
2. To determine boundary layer thickness and displacement thickness.

Apparatus

Wind tunnel (type : open circuit), Prandtl tube, manometer.

Theory

Because of the viscous characteristics of a fluid flowing past a body, the fluid has a tendency to adhere to the body. As a result, 'no slip' conditions prevail and the fluid at the boundary has the same velocity as that of the boundary. The thin zone in the vicinity of boundary, in which the intertial forces are relatively small compared to viscous forces, is termed as the boundary layer.

Consider a fluid flow past a flat plate which is placed parallel to the flow as shown in the figure. At the leading edge, $x = 0$, of the plate, the thickness of the boundary layer zone is zero. Thickness of this zone increases with increase in x. In the initial portion of the flat plate the flow within the boundary layer is laminar and accordingly the boundary layer is termed as laminar boundary layer. After some distance, flow within the boundary layer is, however, turbulent. Such a boundary layer is called turbulent boundary layer. In the turbulent boundary layer zone there still exists a very thin layer near the boundary in which the flow is laminar. This thin layer is called laminar sublayer. In between laminar boundary layer zone and turbulent boundary layer zone there exists a transition zone. Velocity distribution in the laminar boundary layer zone follows parabolic variation while in the turbulent boundary layer zone the velocity variation is logarithmic in nature.

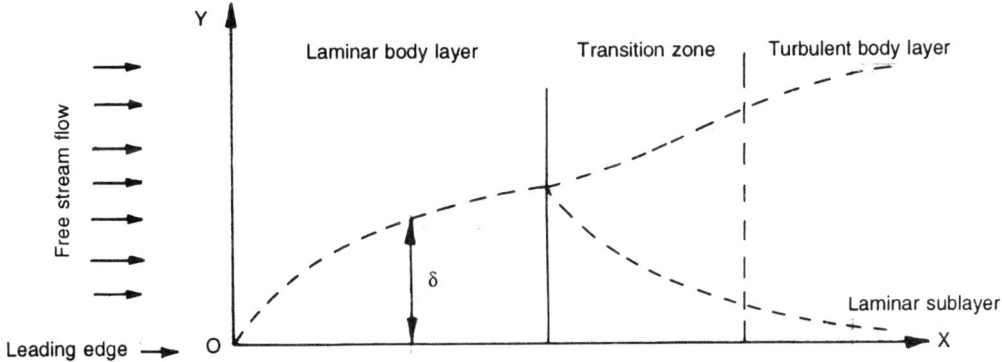

The extent of the viscous effects near a body is measured in terms of a boundary layer thickness. Two commonly used measures are the nominal thickness and the displacement thickness of the boundary layer. The nominal thickness of boundary layer is defined as the value of y at which the velocity offlow is 99% of the free stream velocity. In other words, at $y = \delta$, $v = 0.99v_0$. Here, v represents velocity of flow at any value y, v_0 is the free stream velocity.

Displacement thickness $\delta*$ is defined as the distance by which the boundary should be shifted so that the resulting volume of fluid flowing with uniform velocity distribution is the same as that of the actual flow. Obviously, from the figure,

$$\delta* = \frac{\text{Area ABC}}{v_0}$$

Here, area ABC represents the reduction in flow rate due to boundary layer effects.

Velocity variation in a turbulent boundary layer is given by

$$\frac{v}{v_0} = \left(\frac{v}{\delta}\right)^n$$

in which n varies from 1/7 to 1/10.

Procedure

1. Start the wind tunnel and let the Prandtl tube touch the bottom of the tunnel.
2. Take manometer readings h_1 and h_2.
3. Raise the Prandtl tube by 2 mm and repeat step (2).
4. Repeat step (3) till the centre of the tunnel is reached or when no change in manometer readings is observed for five different successive positions of Prandtl tube.

Observations

Diameter of Prandtl tube, d = ...
Specific weight of manometer liquid, ρ_m = ...
Conversion factor = ...
Initial reading of the pointer gauge = ...
Slope of inclined manometer, $\sin \theta$ = ...
Specific weight of air, ρ_{air} = ...

$C' = \dfrac{\rho_m}{\rho_{air}} - 1 = $ ....

$P_i = $ ....

S. No.	Pointer gauge reading, P_i	Distance from the boundary $y = P_t - P_i + d$	Manometer readings			Velocity, $v = \sqrt{2g\Delta h}$	$\dfrac{v}{v_0}$	$\dfrac{v}{\delta}$
			Limb 1, h_1	Limb 2, h_2	$h = C'(h_1 - h_2)x \sin \theta$			
1.								
2.								
3.								
4.								
5.								
6.								
7.								
8.								
9.								
10.								
11.								
12.								
13.								
14.								
15.								

Calculations

Plot v v/s y on plain graph paper. Determine the free stream velocity. Find out the value of $y(\delta)$ at which $v = 0.99 v_0$.

$$\delta* = \frac{\text{Area ABC}}{v_0}$$

Plot $\dfrac{v}{\delta}$ vs $\dfrac{v}{v_0}$ on log-log graph paper.

Results

      Slope of the line, n = ...

      Body layer thickness = ...

      Displacement thickness = ...

Questions

    1. Why the boundary layer is important and give some practical examples.
    2. If the viscosity of the fluid is increased, what will happen to the thickness of the boundary layer?

Experiment No. 16

Object

To study the flow over a hump placed in an open channel.

Apparatus

It consists of a glass-walled rectangular flume about 6 m long, 0.6 m wide and 0.8 m deep. Two semi-cylindrica wooden humps of about 25 mm and 50 mm radius with flat surface. Pointer gauge scale.

Theory

Let a hump of small height z be placed on the bed of a rectangular channel carrying a discharge Q under uniform flow conditions. The specific energies are E_1 and E_2 at sections 1-1 and 2-2 respectively.

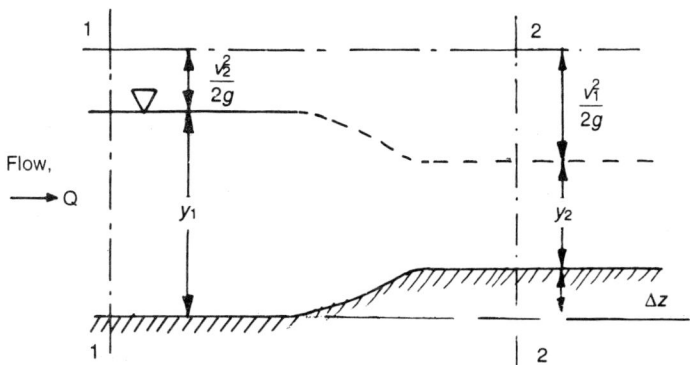

Then
$$E_2 = y_2 + \frac{v_2^2}{2g} = y_2 + \frac{Q^2}{2gBy_2^2}$$

$$E_2 = E_1 - \Delta z^2$$

$$E_1 = y_1 + \frac{v_1^2}{2g} = y_1 + \frac{Q^2}{2gBy_1^2}$$

where y_1 and y_2 are the depths; Q = flow rate; B is the width of channel; v_1 and v_2 are the velocities at section 1-1 and 2-2, respectively. If the critical height is z_c then if Δz exceeds $(\Delta z)_c$, the flow conditions upstream can be modified and the flow conditions over the hump will be that of critical state. New conditions of flow on the upstream of hump will be given as :

$$E_1' = E_c + \Delta z$$

where, E_1' is the new value of E_1.

If $z < (\Delta z)_c$, the upstream conditions remain unaffected. If $z = (\Delta z)_c$, the upstream conditions remain unchanged but the flow over the hump is in critical state. Then,

$$E_2 = E_c = E_1 - (\Delta z)_c$$

Procedure

1. Establish uniform flow at a depth of about 150 mm in the flume by adjusting discharge and the tail gate position.
2. Measure the depth of flow at few sections along the centre line of the flume.
3. Place hump No. 1 on the bed transverse to the flow leaving no gap between the channel bed and the hump.
4. Take pointer gauge readings for water surface and bed elevation at different flow sections upstream and downstream of the hump along the centre line of the flume.
5. Measure the discharge.
6. Replace hump No. 1 by hump No. 2 and repeat steps (4) and (5).

Observations

Sl. No.	y_1	E_1	$E_2 = E_1 - \Delta z$	y_2 from plot	y_2 (observed)
Hump 1					
Hump 2					

Calculations

1. Plot the water surface profile.   2. Plot E vs y curve.

Results

Critical z_c = ...

Questions

1. What do you understand by critical flow? Why it is important?
2. Give some examples of hump in real life situations?

SECTION 4

HIGHWAY LABORATORY

In the highway laboratory the highway materials are tested. The important materials are stone aggregates, bitumen, fine aggregates, cement, etc.

Abrasion test of stone is performed to find out the hardness of stone aggregates. Hardness is the property which resists the continuous abrasion. On the top surface of highway there is continuous abrasion of aggregates so the hard stone aggregates are desired for top surface.

The stone aggregates of the top surface should be tough enough to resist the impact loading. The toughness of stone is nothing but the impact value. So before the use of stone aggregates in top surface their impact value must be determined. Apart from abrasion and impact loading the mutual abrasion also takes place among aggregates which is called attrition. The aggregates used should be round enough to minimise the attrition, otherwise if once attrition has started the packing of aggregates gets disturbed and the top surface is damaged. This attrition value is determined by attrition test. In addition to these properties, the stone aggregates should be strong enough to bear the load. That is, the aggregates should not be crushed under traffic load. This crushing strength is determined by crushing value test in highway laboratory. The flaky stone particles are poor in bearing of load. So the flakiness and elongation index should be found out by standard gauges in the laboratory.

Bitumen is used as the binding material in highway construction. Consistency and durability of bitumen are two very important properties. Consistency gives the penetration value of bitumen, i.e. whether the bitumen is hard or soft. The requirement of the hard or the soft bitumen is dependent upon the temperature of the place where it is going to be used.

Experiment No. 1

Object :

To determine the impact value of aggregates.

Apparatus/Equipment :

Impact testing machine, cylindrical measure, tamping rod, sieves, balances, etc.

Theoretical background :

The property of material to resist impact is toughness. Stone aggregates should be tough enough to resist the pounding action or impact of traffic load.

The aggregate impact value is relative measure of resistance of aggregate to impact or sudden shock. Aggregate impact value is the percentage of the fines formed in terms of total weight of the sample.

$$\text{Aggregate impact value} = \frac{A}{B} \times 100$$

where A = weight of material passing through 2.36 IS sieve.

B = Original weight of sample before the test.

Procedure :

1. Take some aggregates passing through 12.5 mm IS sieve and retained on 10 mm sieve.
2. Fill the cylinder with aggregate in three approximately equal layers by tamping 25 times each layer by tamping rod.
3. Remove the excess aggregate from the top layer by tamping rod as straight edge. Find the weight of test sample.
4. Now transfer the test sample from cylinder to the cup of impact machine which is firmly fixed on the base of the impact machine.
5. Compact the testing sample by tamping (25 strokes).
6. Raise the hammer of the machine until its lower face is 38 cm above the upper surface of aggregate in cup.
7. Allow the hammer to fall freely on aggregate and apply 15 such blows, each being delivered at an interval of not less then one second.
8. Remove the aggregate from cup. Sieve it through 2.36 mm IS sieve. Find the weight of passing material A.

Observations :

Weight of the original sample B =

Weight of the passing material A =

Calculation : Aggregate impact value $I = \dfrac{A}{B} \times 100$

Result : Aggregate impact value =

Experiment No. 2

Object :

To determine the crushing value of stone aggregate.

Apparatus/Equipment :

Cylinder with base plate and plunger, tamping rod, balance, compression testing machine, etc.

Theoretical background :

Aggregates used in pavements are subjected to crushing traffic wheel loads. Aggregates should be strong enough to resist crushing load. The crushing value provide a measure of resistance to crushing under a gradually applied compressive load.

It is defined as the ratio of the weight of the fines (W_2) passing through the specified IS sieve to the total weight of the sample (W_1) expressed as percentage.

$$\text{Aggregate crushing value} = \frac{W_2}{W_1} \times 100$$

Procedure :

1. Select about 1.5 kg. aggregate passing through 12.5 mm sieve and retained on 10 mm sieve.
2. Fill the cylinder by aggregate in three layers of approximately equal depth by tamping each layer 25 times by tamping rod.
3. Level off the top layer by tamping rod as a straight edge.
4. Find the weight of the test sample and place the plunger on the top of the cylinder.
5. Place the cylinder on the compression testing machine. Apply the load at a uniform rate of 4 tonnes per minute until the load reaches to 40 tonnes.
6. Remove the aggregate from cylinder, sieve it through 2.36 mm IS sieve, collect the passing material and weigh it.
7. Repeat the test on second sample of the same weight.

Observations :

	1	2
Total wt. of dry sample (W_1)		
Wt. of fines (W_2)		

Calculations :

Aggregate crushing value $= \dfrac{W_2}{W_1} \times 100$

	1	2
Aggregate crushing value		
Av. Agg. Crushing value		

Result :

Average aggregate crushing value =

Experiment No. 3

Object :

To determine the percentage wear due to dry attrition.

Apparatus/Equipment :

Deval machine, sieve, balance, etc.

Theoretical background :

The wear due to rubbing of similar aggregates against one another is called attrition. Attrition is an indirect measure of hardness. Attrition value is percentage of worn material in terms of total weight.

$$\text{Dry attrition value} = \frac{\text{Weight of material passing through 1.6 mm IS sieve after test}}{\text{Weight of the sample before the test}} \times 100$$

$$\text{Coefficient of wear} = \frac{40}{\text{dry attrition value}}$$

Procedure :

1. Take about 5 kg dry aggregate passing through 50 mm IS sieve and retained on 32.5 mm IS sieve. Place the sample in cylinder of Deval machine and fix the lid.
2. Rotate the machine at the speed of 30 to 33 rpm for 10,000 revolutions. At the end of test, remove the whole test sample from cylinder of machine.
3. Sieve the test sample through 1.6 mm IS sieve and find the weight of the passing material.

Observations :

1. Weight of aggregate specimen before test, W_1 =
2. Weight of material passing through 1.6 mm IS sieve, W_2 =

Calculations :

$$\text{Dry attrition value} = \frac{W_2}{W_1} \times 100$$

$$\text{Coefficient of wear} = \frac{40}{\text{dry attrition value}}$$

Result :

Dry attrition value =
Coefficient of wear =

Experiment No. 4

Object :

To determine the coefficient of hardness or resistance to wear of stone aggregate by

    (a) Los Angeles abrasion test

    (b) Deval abrasion test

    (c) Dorry abrasion test

(a) Los Angeles Test

Apparatus/Equipment :

Los Angeles machine, sieve, etc.

Theoretical background :

The aggregate used in surface course are under constant rubbing or abrasion due to traffic movement. This action may increase further in presence of abrasive material like sand between tyres and aggregate of top surface.

    This test determines the percentage wear due to relative rubbing action between aggregates and steel balls. Steel balls are used as abrasive charge. Pounding action of ball also comes in picture while conducting the experiment.

$$\text{Percentage wear} = \frac{\text{Loss of weight due wear}}{\text{Original weight}} \times 100$$

Procedure :

1. Take some quantity of clean dried aggregates and some steel balls. The weight of aggregates and no. of steel balls depend upon the grading of aggregate. Now put them in cylinder of machine.
2. Rotate the machine at a speed of 30 to 33 rpm for 500 revolutions in case of A, B, C, D grade aggregates and for 1000 revolutions in case of E, F, G grade aggregates.
3. After the desired number of revolutions, stop the machine and remove the material from it.
4. Sieve the material through the IS sieve coarser than 1.7 mm. Now sieve the finer portion further by 1.7 mm IS sieve. Wash and dry the portion of the material coarser than 1.7 mm and weigh it.
5. Repeat the test on aggregates of same grade and find the average percentage wear.

Observations :

    1. Grade of aggregate = _____

    2. No. of spheres used = _____

    3. Weight of charge = _____

Weight of aggregate, W_1 =
Weight of the material coarser than 1.7 mm IS sieve, W_2 =

Calculations :

	1	2
Loss of weight due to wear, $(W_1 - W_2)$		
Percentage wear $= \dfrac{(W_1 - W_2)}{W_1} \times 100$		

Average percentage wear =

Result :

Los Angeles abrasion value = Average percentage wear =

(b) Deval Abrasion Test

Apparatus/Equipment :

Deval machine, balance, etc.

Theoretical background :

Loss of weight by abrasion is the difference between the original weight of test sample (W_1) and weight of material coarser than 1.7 mm (W_2) after the test. The percentage wear is the loss in weight by abrasion expressed as percentage of original weight.

$$\text{Percentage wear} = \frac{W_1 - W_2}{W_1} \times 100$$

Procedure :

1. Find out the grade and specific gravity of material.
2. According to the specific gravity, weigh the desired quantity of aggregate and take the 6 steel balls as abrasive charging.
3. Place the aggregates and balls in machine.
4. Rotate the machine at the speed of 30 to 33 rpm for 10,000 revolutions.
5. After the completion of revolutions discharge the material from machine, sieve it by 1.7 mm IS sieve.
6. Wash and dry the material coarser than 1.7 mm and weigh it.

Observations :

a) Grade of the material =
b) Specific gravity of the material =
c) Weight of material in starting of test (i.e., original weight), W_1 =
d) Weight of material coarser than 1.7 mm after the test, W_2 =

Calculations :

1. Loss of weight due to abrasion, $(W_1 - W_2) =$

2. Percentage wear $= \dfrac{W_1 - W_2}{W_1} \times 100 =$

Result :

Percentage wear =

Grading and abrasive charge specifications for Los Angeles test

Grading	80-63	63-50	50-40	40-25	25-20	20-12.5
A	–	–	–	1250	1250	1250
B	–	–	–	–	–	2500
C	–	–	–	–	–	–
D	–	–	–	–	–	–
E	2500*	2500*	5000*	–	–	–
F	–	–	5000*	500*	–	–
G	–	–	–	5000*	5000*	–

(The table presents grading of aggregates for Deval abrasion test.)

Weight of sample for Deval abrasion test.

* 2% tolerance.

(c) Dorry's Abrasion Test

Apparatus/Equipment :

Dorry's machine, stone specimen, balance, etc.

Theoretical background :

In this test the stone specimen is rubbed on metal disc in presence of sand as absorbing agent. Coefficient of hardness (h) of stone is given by the following equation.

$$h = \frac{20 - \text{loss of weight in grams}}{3}$$

Procedure :

1. Place the cylindrical specimen of stone in the holder of Dorry's machine with its axis vertical and apply specified load of 1250 gms.
2. Revolve the disc of machine at the speed of 28 rpm for 1,000 revolutions. During this period feed the dry standard sand continuously through funnel.
3. After the completion of revolutions remove the specimen from holder, clean it and weigh it.

Observations :

    a) Original weight of cylindrical specimen, W_1 =

    b) Weight of worn specimen after test, W_2 =

Calculation :

    Loss of weight in gms = $W_1 - W_2$ =

$$h = 20 - \frac{W_1 - W_2}{3}$$

Result :

    Coefficient of hardness, h =

Experiment No. 5

Object :

To determine the flakiness index and elongation index.

Apparatus/Equipment :

Balance, sieve (63, 50, 40, 31.5, 25, 20, 16, 12.6, 10, 6.13 mm), shaker, etc.

Theoretical background :

Flakiness index of aggregates is the percentage by weight of particles whose least dimension (thickness) is less than three fifth of their mean dimension. Mean dimension is the average size of aggregates. The test is applicable to sizes larger than 6.3 mm.

$$\text{Flakiness index} = \frac{\text{Weight of material passing through thickness gauge}}{\text{Total weight of aggregate}}$$

Elongation index of aggregates is the percentage by weight of particles whose greatest dimension (length) is greater than one and four fifth (1.8) times their mean dimension. This test is applicable to sizes larger than 6.3 mm.

$$\text{Elongation index} = \frac{\text{Weight of material retained by length gauge}}{\text{Total weight}} \times 100$$

Flakiness Index

Procedure :

1. Take some aggregates and sieve them properly through the sieve set (63 mm to 6.3 mm in descending order). The taken quantity must be sufficient to provide minimum 200 sieved pieces for test.
2. Separate the aggregates by their sizes and find the weight of aggregate of each size, (W_i).
3. Try to pass each aggregate through corresponding slot in the thickness gauge.
4. Weigh all the pieces which passes through the particular slot.

Calculations :

a) Total weight of material, $W = W_1 + W_2 + W_3 + \ldots =$

b) Weight of material passing through thickness gauge, $w =$

c) Flakiness index $= \dfrac{w}{W} \times 100$

Result : Flakiness index of aggregates =

Elongation Index

Procedure :

1. Sieve the aggregates through the sieve set and determine the weight of aggregates of each size separately, (W_i).
2. Try to pass each piece through corresponding gauge size.
3. Weigh all the material retained by length gauge.

Observation :   (A)

S. No.	Passing IS sieve	Retained on IS sieve	Thickness of slot, mm	Wt. of material of corresponding size, W_1	Weight of material passing through, W_i
1.	63	50	33.9		
2.	50	40	27.0		
3.	04	31.5	19.5		
4.	31.5	25	61.95		
5.	25	20	13.5		
6.	20	16	10.8		
7.	16	12.5	8.56		
8.	12.5	10	6.75		
9.	10	6.3	4.89		

(B)

S. No.	Passing through IS sieve	Retained on IS sieve	Length of gauge	Weight of material	Retained material by length gauge
1.	63	50	–	–	–
2.	50	04	–	–	–
3.	40	31.5	81.0	–	–
4.	31.5	25	–	–	–
5.	25	20	40.5	–	–
6.	20	16	32.4	–	–
7.	16	12.5	25.6	–	–
8.	12.5	10.0	20.2	–	–
9.	10.0	6.3	14.7	–	–

Calculations :

    a) Total weight of material $W = W_1 + W_2 + W_3 + \ldots =$

    b) Weight of material retained by length gauge $w =$

    c) Elongation index $= \dfrac{w}{W} \times 100$

Result :   Elongation index of aggregates =

Experiment No. 6

Object :

To examine the penetration (consistency) of bituminous material.

Apparatus/Equipment :

Penetrometer, thermometer, water bath, stop watch, etc.

Theoretical background :

This test determine the hardness or softness of bituminous material. Higher the penetration value, softer will be the material. Penetration value is the amount of vertical penetration that a standard needle will penetrate through bituminous material under a standard load, at a standard temperature and in standard time period.

Procedure :

1. Melt the sample, stir it and make it homogenous.
2. Pour the sample into container and keep the container in water bath at 25°C for at least one hour.
3. The depth of bituminous material in container should be at least 15 mm more than the expected penetration.
4. Put the container at penetrometer below the needle.
5. Bring the needle of penetrometer in contact with the surface of the test specimen and set the zero reading of needle.
6. Release the needle for five seconds. Note the final reading on dial.
7. Take 5 to 6 readings and find average penetration value.

Observations :

S. No.	Sample	Penetration

Calculation :

$$\text{Average penetration value} = \frac{\text{Penetration value}}{\text{No. of samples}}$$

Result :

Average penetration value =
and, therefore, grade of bituminous material.

Experiment No. 7

Object :

To determine the ductility of bituminous material.

Apparatus/Equipment :

Sample mould, water bath, square and trowel, ductility machine, etc.

Theoretical background :

Ductility is the property of material by which it can be stretched without cracking. Here ductility is expressed as distance in centimeter to which a standard briquette of bitumen can be stretched before the thread breaks. The binder or bituminous material which does not possess sufficient ductility would crack and thus provide pervious pavement surface.

Procedure :

1. Make the bituminous sample a homogenous fluid and pour it in mould. Place the mould on brass plate.
2. After 30 to 40 minutes, place the whole assembly in water bath maintained at 27°C for 20 minutes.
3. Remove the assembly from bath, cut off excess bitumen level and surface by hot knife and place it again in water bath for 85 to 95 minutes.
4. Remove the sides of mould and hook the clips on machine without causing any initial strain and set the pointer at zero.
5. Start the machine to pull the clips horizontally apart. While test is in operation make sure that sample is immersed in water at the depth of at least 10 mm.
6. Record the distance at which bitumen thread breaks.
7. Repeat the test for two more samples of same type of bitumen.

Observations :

a) Weight of sample (same for all samples) =

b) Test temperature (same for all samples) =

c) Grade of bitumen (same for all samples) =

1	2	3

d) Ductility in cm =

Calculation :

Average ductility in cm =

Result :

Ductility value = Average ductility =

Reference for Highway Engineering Laboratory

1. Khanna, S.K. and Justo, C.E.G., Highway Material Testing, Nemchand and Brothers, Roorkee, 3rd edition, 1974.
2. Oglesby, Clarkson H., Highway Engineering, Wiley Eastern Ltd., New York, 3rd edition, 1975.
3. Khanna. S.K., and Justo, C.E.G., Highway Engineering, Nemchand and Brothers, Roorkee, 6th edition, 1987.

SECTION 5

CONCRETE LABORATORY

Properties of cement and concrete are determined in concrete laboratory. The experiments related to determining some important properties of cement and concrete are explained in this chapter.

Normal consistency gives the idea about the quality of selection of cement for a particular project. Fineness modules of cement is related to initial and final setting time of cement. Initial and final setting times decide the work rate of concreting and the curing. Generally the cement having less initial setting time is not desirable since the primary bonds which have been formed are broken away while concreting.

Compressive and tensile strength determination of concrete is very important in design field without knowing the compressive and tensile strength of concrete a concrete structure or any component there of can not be designed. Workability of concrete is also a factor which should be kept in mind while designing. A concrete mix which is strong enough but not workable is not an economic mix. Workability of concrete is the degree of with which concrete mix flows to remote corner of the form work.

Experiment No. 1

Object :

To determine the quantity of water for cement paste for normal consistency.

Apparatus :

Vicat needle apparatus with plunger of 10 mm dia trowel, balance, etc.

Theoretical background :

The percentage of water by weight of cement which produces a consistency which permits plunger having diameter 10 mm. to penetrate up to depth of 5 to 7 mm above the bottom of mould is called the normal consistency of cement paste.

Procedure :

1. Take 400 gm of cement and place it in enamel trough.
2. Add 25% of water in dry cement and mix it. The gauging time should not be less than 3 minutes and not more than 5 minutes. The gauging time is time consumed from adding of water in dry cement to commencing to fill the mould.
3. After mixing properly, fill the Vicat mould with this paste.
4. Level the surface of cement with top of mould.
5. Place the mould on the non porous plate under the plunger of apparatus and adjust the indicator in such a way that it shows zero reading when plunger touches the bottom of mould (i.e., non-porous plate).
6. Release the plunger and note down the reading.
7. If the penetration is less than the desired one then make another trial sample by increasing water content and find the penetration.
8. Repeat the step 7 until the desired penetration, i.e., penetration upto 5 to 7 mm. above the bottom is achieved.

Observations :

S. No.	Quantity of cement	Quantity of water	% of water by weight	Penetration above from bottom

Result : Normal consistency of cement paste =

Experiment No. 2

Object :

To determine the fineness of cement.

Apparatus :

Sieve of 75 microns, balance, etc.

Theoretical background :

This test finds out whether the cement is ground properly or not. Finer cement particle leads to higher rate of hydration and quick development of strength by cement.

Observations :

S. No.	Wt. of cement taken, W	Wt. of cement, W_1, retained on sieve	Percentage of retained, $\frac{W_1}{W} \times 100$
1.			
2.			
3.			

Calculation :

    Average percentage of wt. retained =

Result :

    Cement is/(is not) ground well since percentage of weight retained =
which is/(is not) greater than 10%.

Experiment No. 3

Object :

To determine the initial and final setting time of cement.

Apparatus :

Vicat's needle apparatus, balance, stop watch, etc.

Theoretical background :

Initial setting time is the time consumed from addition of water into dry cement to the instant at which needle of 1 mm^2 section fails to pierce the test sample to a depth of 5 mm from the bottom. Final setting time is time consumed from addition of water into dry cement to the instant at which needle of 1 mm^2 with 5 mm dia attachment makes an impression on the sample but attachment fails to make it.

Procedure :

1. Weigh 400 gm of cement and place it in enamel trough.
2. Add 0.85 P % water by weight of cement and mix it thoroughly, where P is the normal consistency of cement.
3. Fill the mould with cement paste and level off the cement surface with top of mould. The gauging time should not be less than 3 minutes and should not be more than 5 minutes.
4. Place the mould on non porous plate under the needle of apparatus.
5. Bring the needle in contact with the cement surface and release it.
6. Repeat the step (5) after every 2 minutes until the needle fails to pierce the sample for about 5 mm measured from the bottom of the mould note down this time. It is initial setting time.
7. Replace the needle by needle with an annular attachment.
8. Bring the needle with attachment near the surface of cement and release it.
9. Repeat the step (8) until the needle makes an impression on surface and attachment does not make impression.
10. Note down this time also.

Observations :

Quantity of cement =
Normal consistency, P =
Quantity of water =
Initial setting time =
Final setting time =

Calculation : Quantity of water required $= 0.85 \times P \times \dfrac{\text{wt. of cement}}{100} =$

Result : Initial setting time =
Final setting time =

Experiment No. 4

Object :

Determination of tensile and compressive strengths of cement.

a) Tensile strength determination.

Apparatus :

Mould assembly, balance, tension testing m/c, etc.

Theoretical background :

Tensile strength of cement is the measure of ability of cement mortar specimen to withstand in tensile load.

Procedure :

1. Weigh 250 gm of cement, 750 gm of sand and mix them properly.
2. Take (P/5 + 2.5) % water of total weight of sand and cement and mix it in sand and cement. Here P is the normal consistency of cement.
3. Oil the interior surface of mould (which is of briquette shape).
4. Put the mould on table and place the whole quantity of mortar in briquette by compacting it with tamping rod.
5. Put the mould at temp $27 \pm 2°C$ and relative humidity 90% for 24 hrs.
6. At the end of this period remove the specimens from moulds and submerge them in clean and fresh water. This water should be renewed after every week.
7. Take out three specimens and test them after 3 days. Similarly test 3 specimens after 7 days.

Observations :

Cross-sectional area of specimen at failure section =

S. No.	Strength after 3 days	S. No.	Strength after 7 days
1.		1.	
2.		2.	
3.		3.	

Calculations :

Average tensile strength after 3 days =

Average tensile strength after 7 days =

Result :

Tensile strength of cement =

b) Compressive strength determination

Apparatus :

Mould, balance, vibrator, compression testing m/c, etc.

Theoretical background :

Compressive strength of cement is the measure of ability of cement mortar specimen to withstand the compressive load. It enables to distinguish rapid hardening cement from low heat and ordinary cement.

Procedure :

1. Weigh 185 gm of cement, 555 gm of sand and mix them properly.
2. Take (P/4 + 3) % water of total weight of cement and sand mix it in cement and sand. P is normal consistency of cement. The quantities taken are for one specimen only. Material for each specimen should be mixed separately according to above mentioned quantities.
3. Oil the interior surfaces of the mould.
4. Place each mould on vibrator and fill them with cement sand mix by vibrating.
5. Keep the moulds (cubes) at temp $27 \pm 2°C$ and in 90% relative humidity for 24 hrs.
6. At the end of this period remove the specimens from moulds and place them in clean water.
7. Test the cubes after 7 days and find the compressive strength of cement. This time period of 7 days may change according to quantity of cement.

Observations :

Dimensions of specimen (cube) =

S. No.	Compressive strength of cement = $\dfrac{\text{Load at failure}}{\text{Cross–sectional area}}$
1.	
2.	
3.	

Calculation :

Average compressive strength of cement =

Result :

Compressive strength of cement =

Experiment No. 5

Object :

To determine compressive strength of nominal mix concrete of a given grade.

Apparatus :

Balance, vibrator, cube, mould, etc.

Theory :

Strength of concrete mix varies according to grade of concrete. Proportions of materials for different grade of concrete are given below.

Grade of concrete	Qty of dry agg. per 50% kg of cement	Proportion of fine to coarse aggregate	Qty. of water per 50 kg tub
M 5	800 kg	Lower limit 1 : 5/2	60
M 7.5	625 kg	Upper limit 1 : 3/2 In general 1 : 2	45
M 10	480 kg		34
M 15	350 kg		32
M 20	250 kg		30

The quantities of ingredients required for 1 cubic meter of concrete are calculated from following equation.

$$\frac{1}{1000}\left[\text{water} + \frac{\text{cement (kg)}}{\text{sp. gr. of cement}} + \frac{\text{FA (kg)}}{\text{sp. gr. of FA}} + \frac{\text{CA (kg)}}{\text{sp. gr. of coarse Ag.}} \right] = 1 - 0.02$$

where .02 corresponds 0 to 2% air content.

Procedure :

1. Calculate the quantities of cement, coarse aggregate, fine aggregate, water required for making 6 cubes of desired grade of concrete by eqn. (1). The size of cube is 15 cm.
2. Place the concrete mix in cube and vibrate it. After vibration, level the top surface of cube by removing excess concrete.
3. Put the cube 27 ± 2°C for 24 hrs. After the end of this period remove the concrete cubes from mould and submerge them in water.
4. Determine the compressive strength of three cubes after 7 days and of other three after 28 days of curing.
5. Compare the theoretical and experimental values of compressive strength of concrete mix.

Observations :

S. No.	Strength after 7 days	S. No.	Strength after 28 days
1.		4.	
2.		5.	
3.		6.	

Calculation :

Determine the required quantities of water, cement, coarse aggregate, fine aggregate by equation (1)

Result :

Compressive strength of M ..... grade concrete =

Note : To obtain combined aggregate of a certain fineness modulus from the given materials, the proportion of fine to the combined aggregate by weight is given by

$$P = 100 \times \frac{(A - B)}{(A - C)}$$

P = Proportion of fine to combined aggregate by weight

A = Fineness modulus of coarse aggregate

B = Fineness modulus of combined aggregate

C = Fineness modulus of fine aggregate.

After determining the required quantities of ingredients the steps for mix design are same as explained.

Experiment No. 6

Object :

To determine the modulus of rupture of concrete.

Apparatus :

Vibrating table, mould, balance, etc.

Theoretical background :

Whenever the direct load is applied to a beam, the top fibres are in compression and bottom fibres are in tension. The maximum tensile stress at the bottom fibre of the beam is known as modulus of rupture.

Procedure :

1. Measure the dimensions of beam mould and determine the total volume of it.
2. Select any grade of concrete and according to it, calculate the quantities of cement, coarse aggregate, fine aggregate, water required to make the concrete beam.
3. Mix the cement, fine aggregate, coarse aggregate and water and prepare the concrete of desired grade.
4. Fill the concrete into mould in layers.
5. Compact each layer by means of vibrating table.
6. Keep the mould at temperature $27 \pm 2°C$ for 24 hrs.
7. Remove the specimen from the mould and submerge in water for 7 days.
8. Take out the specimen from water and wipe off excess water from surfaces of beam.
9. Place the specimen in the testing machine in such a way that load will be applied to the upper most surface.
10. Apply load gradually without any shock, at the rate of 180 kg/min.

Observations :

1. Concrete mix =
2. Dimensions of beam =
3. Volume of beam =
4. Weight of beam =
5. Unit weight of beam =
6. Breaking load, P =
7. a = distance between line of fracture and the nearest support =

Calculations :

(i) a =   (*a* should be > 13.3 cm)

Modulus of rupture, $f_b = \dfrac{P \times L}{b \times d^2}$

(ii) If 11.0 cm. $< a <$ 13.3 cm

$$f_b = \frac{3Pa}{bd^2}$$

(iii) If $a <$ 11.0 then discard the results.

Result :

Modulus of rupture, f_b =

Experiment No. 7

Object :

To determine the flexure strength of concrete using pulse velocity of ultrasonic waves.

Apparatus :

Ultrasonic tester UCT 3.

Theoretical background :

The flexure strength (f) can be expressed in terms of dynamic modulus of elasticity (E) as given below :

$$f = 29.3 + 76.9\,E + 6.9\,E^2 \qquad\qquad\qquad ...(1)$$

Dynamic modulus of elasticity (E) is determined by pulse velocity (V) of ultrasonic waves.

$$E = \frac{V^2 \rho\,(1 + \mu)\,(1 - 2\mu)}{(1 - \mu)}$$

It is assumed that $\mu = 0.24$

The presence of cracks of air gaps can be determined easily.

Procedure :

1. Take out the concrete cubes from water and wipe off the surface water from surfaces of cube.
2. Weigh the cube and determine its density.
3. Pass the ultrasonic waves through the cube of concrete and note down the time taken by wave to pass through the cube.

Observations :

Dimension of concrete cube =

Mass of concrete cube =

Density (ρ) =

S. No.	Time (s)	Velocity
1.		
2.		
3.		

Calculations :

$$E = \frac{V^2 \rho\,(1 + \mu)\,(1 - 2\mu)}{(1 - \mu)}$$

$$f = 29.3 + 76.9\,E + 6.9\,E^2$$

Calculation Table :

S. No.	Velocity	E	f	Average flexure strength
1.				
2.				
3.				

Result :

Flexure strength =

Experiment No. 8

Object :

Workability of concrete by various methods.

Theoretical background :

Concrete is said to be workable if it can be easily mixed and easily placed, compacted and finished, i.e., the ease with which concrete mix flows to the remote corner of the form work.

Table : Consistency measurements by various methods (as per ACI Committee 211)

Workability description	Workability measurement		Vee-Bee time (seconds)
	Slump (mm)	Compacting factor (C.F.)	
Extremely dry	–	–	32-18
Very stiff	–	0.70	18-10
Stiff	0-25	0.75	10-5
Stiff plastic	25-50	0.85	5-3
Plastic	75-100	0.90	3-0
Flowing	150-175	0.95	–

Methods :

Workability of concrete may be determined by the following methods.

(A) Compaction Factor Test

Apparatus :

Compacting factor apparatus as per IS : 1199-1959, two trowels, hand scoop, tamping rod, platform weighing machine, graduated cylinder of 1000 ml capacity.

Theoretical background :

It is based upon the definition that workability is the amount of work necessary to achieve full compaction of concrete. Compacting factor test works on a principal of determining the degree of compaction achieved by a standard amount of work by allowing the concrete to fall through a standard height.

Procedure :

1. Weigh the empty cylinder accurately and note down the mass say W_1 kg.
2. Prepare the sample of concrete with given proportions and W/C ratio.
3. Fill the sample of concrete in upper hopper gently and carefully with hand scoop without compacting.
4. Open the trap door so that the concrete falls into the lower hopper.
5. Immediately after the concrete has come to rest, open the trap door of the lower hopper and allow concrete to fall into the cylinder.
6. Remove the excess concrete remaining above the level of the top of the cylinder.
7. Find the weight of partially compacted concrete thus filled in the cylinder say W_2 kg.
8. Refill the cylinder with the same sample of concrete in layers approximately 5 cm, vibrating each layer heavily so as to expel all the air and to obtain full compaction.
9. Clean the outside of cylinder and weigh it again say W kg.

Observations :

		Specimens		
		I	II	III
A.	Weight of cylinder, W_1 kg			
B.	Weight of cylinder + partially compacted cement, W_2 kg			
C.	Weight of partially compacted concrete, $(W_2 - W_1)$ kg			
D.	Weight of fully compacted concrete + cylinder, W_3 kg			
E.	Weight of fully compacted concrete, $(W_3 - W_1)$ kg			
F.	Water-cement ratio			
G.	Proportions of sample			

Calculations :

Compaction factor =

$$\text{Compaction factor, CF} = \frac{W_2 - W_1}{W_3 - W_1}$$

Result :

(B) Vee-Bee Slump Test Time Test

Apparatus :

Vee-Bee apparatus as per IS : 1199-1959, cylinderical container, sheet metal slump cone, standard iron rod, weighing balance, trowels.

Theory :

Unsupported concrete, when it is fresh, will flow to the sides and a sinking in height will take place. This vertical settlement is called slump.

   The time required for complete remoulding (from one shape to another, i.e., from conical to cylinderical) in seconds is considered as the number of Vee-Bee seconds. This test gives an indication of mobility and to some extent of the compatibility of freshly mixed concrete.

Procedure :

1. Place the sheet metal slump cone in the cylindrical container of the consistometer.
2. Fill the concrete in four layers and tamp each layer with twenty five strokes in a uniform manner over the section of the cone. After the top layer has been tamped, struck off the concrete with trowel so that cone is exactly filled.
3. Move the glass disc attached to the swivel arm and adjust the glass disc. So as to touch the top of the concrete cone and note the initial reading on the graduated rod.
4. Remove the cone from the concrete immediately by raising it in the vertical direction. Lower the transparent disc on the top of the concrete and note down the reading on graduated rod.
5. Switch on the electrical vibrator and start the stop watch. The vibrations are continued until the concrete is remoulded i.e. the surface become horizontal.
6. Record the time required for complete remoulding in seconds which measures the workability as number of Vee-Bee seconds.

Observations and Calculations :

		Specimen		
		I	II	III
A.	Water-cement ratio			
B.	Initial reading on the graduated rod, x_1			
C.	Final reading on the graduated rod, x_2			
D.	Slump, $(x_2 - x_1)$ mm			
E.	Time for complete remoulding, seconds			

Results :

   According to slump test concrete mix is _____

   According to Vee-Bee time concrete mix is _____

(C) Flow Table Method

Theoretical background :

The test determines the fluidity or consistency of concrete by means of flow table. The spread of concrete subjected to jolting is taken as the measure of flow or consistency of concrete.

Apparatus :

Flow table as per IS : 15-1959, mould in the form a frustrum of cone, weighing balance, tamping rod, calipers.

Procedure :

1. Clean the table top and inside of the mould.
2. Centre the mould on the table platform and hold it firmly in place.
3. Fill the mould in two equal layers. Each layer is given 25 strokes with the standard tamping rod in a uniform manner over the cross-section of the mould.
4. After the top layer has been tamped, struck off the surface with a trowel so that the mould is exactly filled. Clean the outside of the mould and table.
5. Remove the mould immediately by lifting it vertically by a steady upward pull.
6. Turn the handle 15 times at the rate of 1 revolution per second so that the concrete has been given a jolt by raising and dropping by 12.5 mm.
7. Measure the diameter of the spread concrete.
8. Obtain the flow or the consistency of concrete by expressing the increase in diameter of concrete specimen as the percentage of the original diameter of 250 mm.

Observations :

		Specimen		
		I	II	III
A.	Base diameter (250 mm)			
B.	Spread diameter (mm)			
C.	Increase in diameter (mm)			

Calculations :

$$\text{Flow per cent} = \frac{\text{increase in dia} \times 100}{\text{original dia}}$$

Result :

The flow of concrete is .... per cent.

Experiment No. 9

Object :

To determine the split tensile strength of concrete of given mix proportions.

Apparatus :

Compression testing machine of sufficient capacity and with an arrangement for applying the load at the specified rate. The bearing faces of both plates shall provide a minimum loading area of 12 mm × the length of the cylinder so that the load is applied over the entire length of the specimen; two packing strips of plywood conforming to IS : 303-1970 for each specimen. The strips shall be 12 mm wide and 3 mm thick and used once only; cylinder moulds of 150 mm diameter and 320 mm height; weighing machine; mixer; tamping rods.

Theoretical background :

The magnitude of tensile stress developed due to the application of compressive load is given by

$$S = \frac{2P}{\pi dl}$$

P = applied load

d = diameter of cylindrical specimen

l = length of cylindrical specimen.

Diameter should be larger than four times the maximum size of coarse aggregate or 150 mm whichever is greater. The length of the specimen should not be less than the diameter and should not be more than twice the diameter.

Procedure :

1. Take the concrete mix used for workability tests.
2. Fill the cylinder mould with four layers, each of approximately 75 mm and tamp each layer more than 35 times with evenly distributed strokes.
3. Remove the surplus concrete from the top of the moulds with the help of a trowel.
4. Cover the moulds with wet mats and put the identification marks after about 3 to 4 hours.
5. Remove the specimens from the moulds after 24 hours and immerse them in water for the final curing. The tests are usually conducted at the ages of 7 and 28 days. The age shall be calculated from the time of addition of water to the dry ingredients.
6. Test at least three specimens for each age of test as follows :
   - iii) Draw diametrical lines on two ends of the specimen so that they are in the same axial plane.
   - ii) Determine the diameter of the specimen to the nearest 0.2 mm by averaging the diameters of the specimen lying in the plane of premarked lines measured near the ends and the middle of the specimen. The length of the specimen also shall be taken to the nearest 0.2 mm by averaging the two lengths measured in the plane containing the premarked lines.
   - iii) Center one of the plywood strips along the centre of the lower plate place the specimen on the

plywood strip and align it so that the lines marked on the end of the specimen are vertical and centered over the plywood strip. The second plywood strip is placed lengthwise on the cylinder centred on the lines marked on the ends of the cylinder. The assembly is positioned to ensure that the lines marked on the ends of the specimen are vertical and the projection of the plane passing through these two lines intersect the centre of the plate.

7. Apply the load without shock and increase it continuously at a rate to produce a splitting tensile stress of approximately 1.4 to 2.1 N/mm^2/min., until no greater load can be sustained. Record the maximum load applied to the specimen.

8. Note the appearance of concrete and any unusual feature in the type of failure.

9. Compute the splitting strength of the specimen to the nearest 0.05 N/mm^2.

Observations :

Identification mark and the date of test	
Age of the specimen at the date of test	
Mass of specimen in kg	
Maximum load, N	
Diameter of the specimen in mm	
Length of the specimen in mm	

Calculation :

$$\text{Tensile stress} = \frac{2P}{\pi dl} = \frac{0.537\,P}{dl}$$

Result :

Tensile strength =

Experiment No. 10

Object :

To determine the percentage bulking of the fine aggregate.

Apparatus :

Balance, measuring cylinder, tamping rod, etc.

Theoritical background :

Whenever water is added to dry sand or it is absorbed from the atmosphere, its volume increases. This increase in volume due to water is known as bulking of sand. It is the ratio of increase in volume to original volume.

Let W_1 be the unit weight of dry compacted sand,

W_2 be the weight of dry sand in m^3, and

W_3 be the unit weight of wet loose sand.

Vol. of one mass unit of dry compacted sand $= \dfrac{1}{W_1}$

Vol. of one mass unit of dry loose sand in wet sand $= \dfrac{1}{W_2}$

Increase in vol. $= \dfrac{1}{W_2} - \dfrac{1}{W_1} = \dfrac{W_1 - W_2}{W_1 W_2}$

Original volume of one mass unit $= \dfrac{1}{W_1}$

$$\% \text{ bulking} = \frac{(W_1 - W_2)/W_1 W_2}{1/W_1} \times 100 = \frac{W_1 - W_2}{W_2} \times 100 \qquad \text{...(1)}$$

Let x % water is added, then $W_3 = W_2 + \dfrac{x}{100} W_2$

$$W_2 = \frac{W_3}{1 + x/100} \qquad \text{...(2)}$$

Procedure :

1. Weigh the empty measuring cylinder.
2. Fill it with dry sand without compacting, level the top surface by striking off the excess sand. Weigh it and find unit weight of dry loose sand.
3. Fill the cylinder by tamping the sand in three equal layer applying 25 strokes on each layer with tamping rod. Weigh it and find out unit weight of dry compacted sand.
4. Take about 6 litres of dry sand and add 2% water by weight of dry sand and mix it properly. Now fill the sand in cylinder with tamping. Weigh it and find out unit weight of wet loose sand and also unit weight of dry loose sand in wet loose sand.
5. Now add 2% more water by weight of dry sand mix it thoroughly. Fill the sand in cylinder and find

out unit weight of dry and wet loose sand. Each time add 2% water and find out unit weight until water content reaches to 20%.

6. Fill the cylinder with water, weigh it and determine the weight of water in cylinder. Thus find the volume of cylinder.

Observations :

1. Wt. of empty cylinder =
2. Wt. of cylinder filled with water =
3. Wt. of cylinder filled with dry loose sand =
4. Wt. of cylinder filled with wet compacted sand =
5. Wt. of sand (about 6 litres) =

S. No.	% of water	Weight of loose wet sand in cylinder	Unit weight of wet sand, W_3	$W_2 = \dfrac{W_3}{1 + \dfrac{x}{100}}$
1.	2			
2.	4			
3.	6			
4.	8			
5.	10			
6.	12			
7.	14			
8.	16			
9.	18			
10.	20			

Calculations :

$$\text{Vol. of cylinder} = \frac{\text{Wt. of water}}{\text{Density of water}}$$

$$\text{Unit Wt. of compacted dry sand, } W_1 = \frac{\text{Wt. of dry compacted sand}}{\text{Vol. of cylinder}}$$

S. No.	% water	W_2	% Bulking = $\dfrac{(W_1 - W_2) \times 100}{W_2}$	Bulking factor = $\dfrac{W_1}{W_2} \times 100$
1.	2			
2.	4			
3.	6			
4.	8			
5.	10			
6.	12			
7.	14			
8.	16			
9.	18			
10.	20			

Result :

Plot a graph between % bulking and water content and find out the water content corresponding to maximum bulking.

Water content at maximum bulking =

Experiment No. 11

Object

To determine soundness of given cement by Le Chatelier method.

Apparatus

'Le-Chatelier' apparatus, two glass plates, temperature controlled water-bath, china dish, balance, graduated cylinder, trowel and IS : 850 micron sieve.

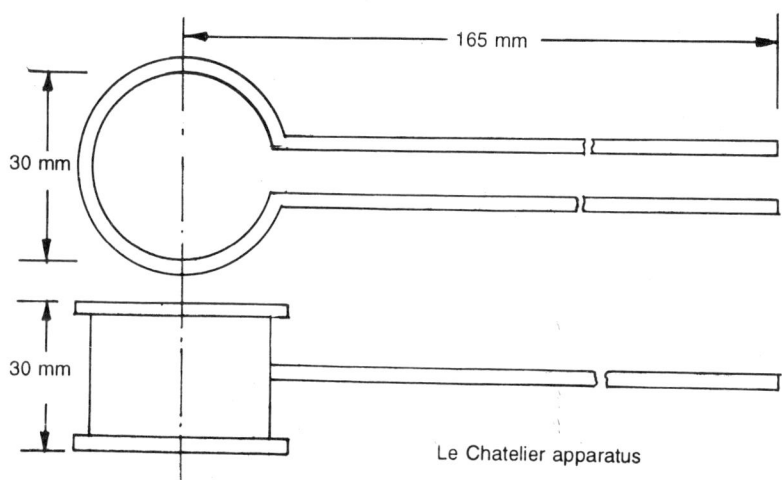

Le Chatelier apparatus

Theory

Excess of free lime and magnesia present in cement slake very slowly and cause appreciable change in volume after setting. In consequence cracks, distortion and distegration result, thereby giving passage to water and atmospheric gases which may have injurious effect on concrete and reinforcement. This defect is known as unsoundness. The expansion is prevented by limiting the quantities of free lime and magnesia in cement.

Procedure

1. Weigh 100 gm of cement. Make a paste of standard consistency.
2. Place the Le Chatelier apparatus on a glass plate and fill it with the paste, and level the top surface.
3. Cover the mould with another piece of glass sheet. Place a small weight on this covering glass-sheet and immediately submerge the whole assembly in water at a temperature of 27°C to 32°C and keep there for 24 hours.
4. Measure the distance between the indicator points after 24 hours and again submerge the mould in water at the temperature prescribed above.
5. Bring the water to boiling point in 25 to 30 minutes and keep it boiling for 3 hours.
6. Remove the mould from the water, allow it to cool and measure the distance between indicator points.
7. The difference between the two measurements gives the expansion of cement and it should not be more than 10 mm according to IS specifications.

Observations

For soundness of cement.

Sl. No.	Initial distance d_1	Final distance d_2	Cement expansion $(d_2 - d_1)$
1.			
2.			
3.			
4.			

Results

An expansion of cement = ...
The cement is/is not sound.

Questions

1. Define soundness of the cement.
2. If the cement is not sound what are the problems a structure feels?
3. What are the measures you should take to remove the effects of unsound cements?

Experiment No. 12

Object

To determine the effect of w/c ratio on the strength of concrete with a given proportion of fine and coarse aggregate (1 : 2.5 by weight) and with a constant slump of 4 cm.

Apparatus

Slump cone apparatus, buckets, trowels, graduated cylinder, balance, tamping rod (15 cm diameter, 60 cm long), universal testing machine, cube modulus of 15 cm size and non-porous plate.

Theory

The concrete of uniform quality can be produced by controlling the workability by varying the w/c ratio. If the grading of the aggregates remains constant, the variation in water content to give constant workability will effectively control the w/c ratio. Hence, this test is based on the principle that concrete having more cement paste in relation to total surface area is more workable.

Procedure

1. Weigh the sand and gravel in the ratio 1 : 2.5. The materials required are 20 kg of gravel and 8 kg of sand for making three 15 cm cubes.
2. Prepare cement slurry with given w/c ratio in the bucket and note the weight of the bucket.
3. Test the mix for slump and increase the amount of slurry until required slump is obtained.
4. Weigh the bucket and find the quantity of cement used.
5. Prepare 15 cm cubes three in number.
6. Test the cubes in compression after 28 days.
7. Repeat the above procedure with cement slurry of different w/c ratios.
8. Calculate the average compressive strength.

Observations

Si. No.	W/c ratio	Specimen number	Average load	Compressive strength
1		1		
		2		
		3		
2		1		
		2		
		3		
3		1		
		2		
		3		
4		1		
		2		
		3		

Results

Questions

1. Why water cement ratio is important? What are the problems you face during construction if w/c ratio is not proper?
2. Can we use any other fluid instead of water and why?

Experiment No. 13

Object

To determine the effect of curing conditions upon compressive strength of (1 : 3) Portland cement mortars.

Apparatus

Compression testing machine, balance moulds, measuring cylinder, trowels, non-porous plate and vibrating table.

Procedure

1. Calculate the materials required for moulds :
   Cement = 185 gm
   Sand = 555 gm
   Water, $\left(\dfrac{P}{4} + 3.5\right)$ percent of aggregate = 81.5 gm.
2. In the mixing crucible, place the mixture of cement and sand in the proportion of 1 : 3 and mix it with water.
3. Place the assembled moulds on the table of the vibrating machine.

4. Immediately, after mixing the mortar, fill the cube moulds in 3 equal layers, tamping each layer 25 times.
5. Keep three specimens in sun, three under any colour paper, three in shade and three in water for effecting different conditions of curing.
6. Test all the specimens at the age of 21 days.

Observations and Calculations

Curing conditions	Specimen No.	Load	Average strength	Time of breaking in seconds	Rate of loading
Sun dried Temperature =	1				
	2				
	3				
Air dried Temperature =	4				
	5				
	6				
Water cured Temperature =	7				
	8				
	9				
Any other					

Precautions

1. The mortar shall not be compressed into the mould with hand.
2. Neglect the results which fall outside by 15 percent of the average results on either side.
3. Cubes should be tested on their sides, not on their faces.
4. The inside of the cube moulds should be oiled to prevent the mortar from adhering to the sides of the moulds.

Effect of rate of loading

The more rapid the static loading of concrete, higher the observed strength. The loading in hydraulic machine is to be applied at a constant rate within the range of 1.5 $kg/cm^2/sec$ to 3.5 $kg/cm^2/sec$, normally 2.5 $kg/cm^2/sec$, is employed.

Results

The best curing condition is .... out of
1.
2.
3.
4.

Questions

1. What do you mean by curing? Why it is important?
2. Can you go for steam curing in real life and how?

Reference for Concrete Laboratory

1. Akyord, Thomas Norman Westhead, Concrete : Properties and Manufacture, Pergamon Press, New York, 3rd edition, 1962.
2. American Concrete Institute, Committee on Reinforced Concrete, Reinforced Concrete Design Handbook, reported by ACI Committee No. 317, Detroit, Michigan, 3rd edition, 1965.
3. Indian Standard Institute for Plain and Reinforced Concrete, (IS : 456-1978), New Delhi.
4. Krishna, Jai and Jain, O.P., Plain and Reinforced Concrete, Nemchand and Brothers, 7th revised and enlarged edition, 1968.
5. Johnson, Roger Paul, Structureal Concrete, McGraw Hill Book Co. Ltd., London, 2nd edition, 1967.
6. Kulkarni, P.D. Ghosh, R.K. and Phull, Y.R., Text Book of Concrete Technology, Oxford and IBH Press, New Delhi, 2nd edition, 1983.
7. Meintosh, John Douglas, Concrete Mix Design, Cement and Concrete Association, London, 2nd edition, 1948.
8. Murdock, Leonard John, Concrete Material and Practice, Arnold Press, London, 5th edition, 1979.
9. Basic Concrete Construction Practices, Portland Cement Association, Wiley Eastern Ltd., New York, 1975.
10. Whitehurst, E.A., Evaluation of Concrete Properties from Sonic Tests, American Concrete Institute, Iowa State University Press, Detroit, Michigan, 1966.
11. Fintel Mark, Handbook of Concrete Engineering, Van Nostrand Press, Reinhold, New York, 1974.
12. Waddell, Joseph J., Concrete Construction Handbook, McGraw Hill Publishing Co. Ltd., New York, 2nd edition, 1968.
13. Kulkarni P.D. and Mittal L.N., Laboratory Institute, Chandigarh.
14. Punmia, Dr. B.C., Reinforced Concrete Structure, Vol. 1, Standard Publishers and Distributors, New Delhi, 4th edition, 1985.
15. Ramamurtham S., Design of Reinforced Concrete Structures, Dhanpat Rai and Sons, Delhi, 10th edition reprinted, 1985.

CHAPTER 6

STRUCTURE LABORATORY

The behaviour of various structures under the action of loads are studied in structure laboratory. The experiments in this chapter covers almost all the important structures.

Three hinged and two hinged arches experiments are performed to determine the maximum load that a particular arch can sustain. Apart from the maximum load position, horizontal thrust, deformation and type of failure are also found out from these experiments. These arches are generally used in doors and gate frames, bridges.

Deformation of beams is determined by Maxwell Betti's law verification. This experiment gives the maximum permissible load for a beam for certian deformation. Without knowing the maximum permissible load a beam cannot be designed.

Euler's law verification reveals the behaviour of struts under the application of load for different end conditions. This law is used in determining the maximum load and effective length of column and hence it is useful in designing the columns.

Experiment No. 1

Object :

To verify Bettimaxwell law.

Apparatus :

A mild steel beam of 100 cm effective span and say 106 cm overall length, equipment for the measurement of deflections.

Theoritical background :

Maxwell's law of reciprocal deflections states : In any structure, the material of which is elastic and obeys Hooke's law and in which the supports are unyielding and the temperature constant, the deflection of point *a* in the direction ab due to a load *P* acting in the diretion cd is numerically equal to the deflection of point *c* in the direction cd due to a load P acting in the direction ab.

This reciprocal relationship exists likewise between rotations produced by a couple and also between the deflection produced by a couple of *P* and rotation produced by a force *P*. Therefore,

$$\delta_{ab} = \delta_{cd}$$

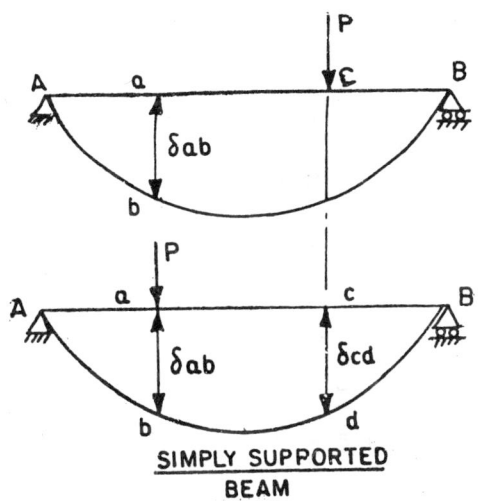

SIMPLY SUPPORTED
BEAM

Procedure :

1. Apply a load (1 kg to 2 kg) at any section of the beam (say X), preferably at or in the middle 1/3rd span of simply supported span or at the end of the cantiliver end in case of a cantilever span so that the deflection may be appreciable.
2. Measure the elevation of the lower edge of the beam at 10 cm intervals by means of a dial guage, cathetometer or a theodolite before and after loading and determine the deflections at 10 cm intervals.
3. Move the same load along the beam by 10 cm and for each position of the load, determine the deflection of the section at which the load was placed initially in step (1).

(Observations table on next page)

Result :

Compare columns (4) and (8). Plot two deflection curves on the same horizontal base and an exaggarated vertical scale and study the curves.

Observations :

Position of Load

Distance from centre of support (cm)	Load at section X				Load moving along the space			
	Beam unloaded (dial guage reading)	Beam loaded (dial gauge reading)	Deflection of various points	Distance from centre of support (cm) load position	Beam unloaded (dial guage reading at X)	Beam loaded (dial gauge reading)	Deflection at section X
(1)	(2)	(3)	(4)	(5)	(6)	(7)	(8)
10							
20							
30							
40							
50							
60							
70							
80							
90							
100							
110							
120							
130							
140							
150							

Experiment No. 2

Object :

To determine the flexual rigidity (EI) of a given beam.

Apparatus :

A steel beam, weights, 4 dial guages, scale.

Theoritical background :

For the beam with two equal overhangs and subjected to two concentracted loads each at the free ends, the maximum deflection y at the centre is given by the following formula

$$y = \frac{WaL^2}{8EI} \qquad ...(1)$$

where

    W = concentrated load at each free end

    a = length of overhang an each side

    L = simply supported span

    E = Young's Modulus of elasticity of the material of the beam

    I = moment of inertia of the cross-section of the beam

    $= \dfrac{bd^3}{12}$ for rectangular cross-section

    b = width of beam section

    d = depth of the beam

    Equation (1) can be written as,

$$EI = \frac{w \cdot a \cdot L^2}{8y} \qquad ...(2)$$

In equation (2), W, a, L and y will be known and EI can be calculated.

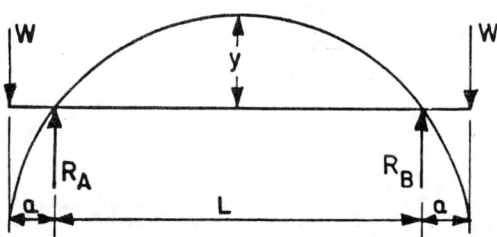

Procedure :

Apply two concentrated loads each of 1 kg at the free ends, measure the central deflection y accurately.

Observations :

       Simply supported span length, L =

       Overhang length on each side =

       Width of beam, b =

       Depth of beam, d =

       Young's modulus of elasticity of beam material =

S. No.	Load	Deflection y in cm
1.	1 kg	
2.	1 kg	
3.	1 kg	

Calculation :

       Moment of inertia of cross-section of the beam = $\dfrac{bd^3}{12}$

       Actual value of $EI = \dfrac{E \times bd^3}{12}$

S. No.	Deflection y	Load W	Experimental value of $EI = \dfrac{W.a.L^2}{8y}$
1.			
2.			
3.			

Result :

Compare the actual value of *EI* to the average of experimental value of *EI*.

Experiment No. 3

Object :

To verify Moment-Area theorems for slopes and deflections of a beam.

Apparatus :

A steel beam, weights, scale, dial guages for measuring deflections.

Theoretical background :

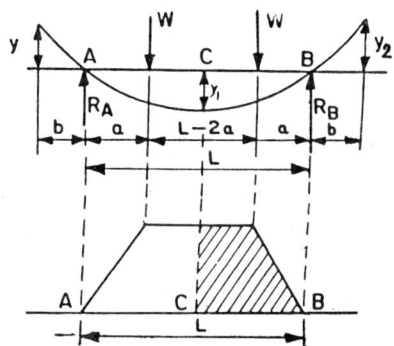

Verification of slopes and deflections

According to moment area theorems :
1. The range of slope of the tangents of the elastic curve between two points A and B is equal to the area under the *M/EI* curve or curvature diagram between these two points.
2. The deflection of point B on the elastic curve from the tangent to this curve at point A is equal to the moment about point B of the area under the *M/EI* curve between the two points A and B.

Slope at B $= \dfrac{y_2}{b}$

$\theta_B - \theta_C$ = Area of *M/EI* curve between C and B

Since the tangent at C is horizontal

$\theta_C = 0$

θ_B = Area of *M/EI* curve between C and B

$= \dfrac{\text{Moment of shaded area about B}}{\text{EI}}$

Procedure :

1. Take a beam of some convenient span L, with two overhang lengths of b each.

2. Load the beam with two equal concentrated loads of W, (say $W = 1$ kg) applied equidistant from A and B. The beam will deflect as shown in figure.

3. Measure the central deflection y_1, and the deflection y_2 at the free end.

Observations :

B =   L =   a =

S. No.	Load at each hanger (kg)	Central deflection, y_1 (cm)	Deflection at free end, y_2 (cm)
1.	1 kg		
2.	1 kg		
3.	1 kg		

Calculations :

S. No.	Load	Slope at B $= \dfrac{y_2}{b}$	Area of curve between c and b	y_1 = def. of b w.r.t. tangent a at c	Moment of area of $\dfrac{M}{EI}$ curve between C and B about B
1.	1 kg				
2.	1 kg				
3.	1 kg				

Result :

i) Slope at B =

ii) Area of $\dfrac{M}{EI}$ curve between C and B

iii) y_1 = def. of B w.r.t. tangent at C =

iv) Moment of an area about B of $\dfrac{M}{EI}$ curve between C and B.

Experiment No. 4

Object :

To study the behaviour of different types of struts.

Apparatus :

Strut model, weights, graph paper, etc.
   The apparatus consists of four struts with the following end conditions :
   a) Both ends hinged.
   b) Both ends fixed.
   c) One end hinged and the other end fixed.
   d) One end fixed and the other completely free. The struts are made of steel strip 10 mm × 0.50 mm.

Theoritical background :

Euler's formula for an axially loaded strut is given by :

$$P_c = \frac{\pi^2 EL}{(L_{eff})^2}$$

where
   P_c = Euler's buckling load
   E = Young's modulus of elasticity of the material of the column
   I = moment of inertia of the cross-section of the column
   L_{eff} = effective length of the column
   L = length of column and is to be taken equal to
         (i) L for both ends hinged;
         (ii) $L/2$ for both ends fixed;
         (iii) $L/\sqrt{2}$ for one end hinged and other end fixed;
         (iv) $2L$ for one end fixed and other end completely free.
   Euler's equivalent lengths may also be found by drawing out the deflected shape of the struts and marking the points of inflection.

Procedure :

   1. Calculate the Euler's buckling load for the strut with both ends hinged.
   2. Grease the rollers of strut. Here top end is fixed and bottom end is completely free, i.e., on rollers.
   3. Place the weights on top of all the struts and note the loads at which they buckle. Tap the bar lightly when loading the model.
   4. Fix a graph paper on the wooden frame behind the struts.
   5. Mark the deflected shape of the struts on the graph paper, with a sharp pencil. Also mark the points of inflection on the deflected curves of the struts and measure the equivalent lengths.

Observations :

Width of strut (mm), b =

Thickness of strut (m), t =

Length of column, L =

S. No.	Type of strut	L_{eff} (measured)	L_{eff} (theoretical)	Euler's buckling load (measured)	Euler's buckling load (theoretical)
1.	Both ends pinned		L		
2.	Both ends fixed		$\dfrac{L}{2}$		
3.	One end pinned and other end fixed		$\dfrac{L}{\sqrt{2}}$		
4.	One end fixed other end free		$2L$		

Calculation :

Moment of inertia = $\dfrac{bt^3}{12}$

S. No.	End condition	Euler's buckling load
1.	Both fixed	$\dfrac{4EI}{L^2}$
2.	One hinged, one fixed	$\dfrac{2EI}{L^2}$
3.	One fixed, one free	$\dfrac{2EI}{4L^2}$
4.	Both ends hinged	$\dfrac{2EI}{L^2}$

Result :

Compare the effective lengths as obtained from actual measurements and theory.

Experiment No. 5

Object :

To determine experimentally and analytically the loads in the three suspension rods supporting an elastic beam with a concentrated load hung midway between two of the suspension rods when :

    i)   the suspension rods are attached at their upper and the rigid supports;

    ii)   the upper end of the central rod is attached to the centre of a similar elastic beam.

Apparatus :

Elasticity coupled beam model, weights, etc.

Theoritical background :

Let the internal forces in the three rods AD, BE and CF be R_1, R_2 and R_3 respectively.

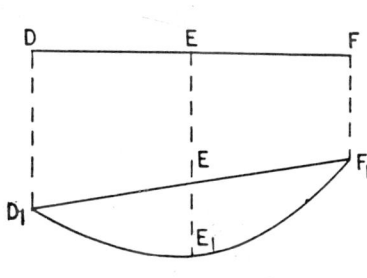 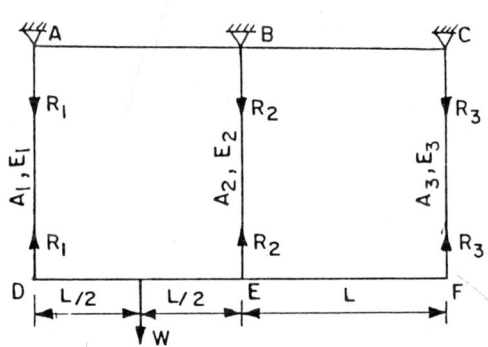

Lengths AD = BE = CF = L

I = Moment of inertia of the cross-section of the beam ABC and the beam DEF

E = Young's modulus of elasticity of the mateial of the beam ABC and beam DEF

E_1, E_2 and E_3 = Modulus of elasticity of the material of rods AD, BE and CF respectively

A_1, A_2 and A_3 = cross-sectional area of rods AD, BE and CF respectively.

$DD_1 = y_1$

$$EE_2 = \frac{y_1 + y_3}{2}$$

$EF_1 = y_2; \quad EF_1 = y_3$

$$E_2E_1 = \frac{11}{96}\frac{WL^3}{EI} - \frac{R_2L^3}{6EI}$$

Case 1 :

When support B exists, beam ABC becomes inoperative. The central deflection at point E of beam DEF, due to load at C and upward R_2 at E, relative to the deflected portions of points D and F given by

$$E = \frac{11}{96} \frac{WL^3}{EI} - \frac{RL^3}{6E^2L} \qquad \text{...(1)}$$

Let y_1 and y_3 be the elongations of the rod AD and point E relative its original position is

$$\frac{y_1 + y_3}{2} + \frac{11}{96} \frac{WL^3}{EI} - \frac{R_2L^3}{6EL} \qquad \text{...(2)}$$

and this should be equal to the elongation of the rod BE, i.e., equal to y_2.

Now $y_1 = \dfrac{R_1L}{A_1E_1}$ $y_2 = \dfrac{R_2L}{A_2E_2}$ and $y_3 = \dfrac{R_3L}{A_3E_3}$

Substituting the values of y_1 and y_3 in eqn. 2

$$\frac{R_2L}{A_2E_2} = \frac{1}{2} \frac{R_1L + R_3L}{A_1E_1} \frac{11}{96} \frac{WL^3}{EI} - \frac{R_2L^3}{6E!} \qquad \text{...(3)}$$

Also $R_1 + R_2 + R_3 = W$ \qquad ...(4)

Taking moments of all the forces about F

$R_1.2L - W\,(\tfrac{3}{2})\,L + R_2.L = 0$

or, $R_1 = \dfrac{3}{4} w - \dfrac{R_2}{2}$ \qquad ...(5)

Solving eqns. (3) (4) and (5) simultaneously for R_1, R_2 and R_3, we obtain

$$R_2 = \frac{W}{2} \times \frac{3K_1 + K_3 + \dfrac{11}{12} \dfrac{L^3}{EI}}{K_1 + 4K_2 + K_3 + \dfrac{2}{3} \dfrac{L^3}{EI}} \qquad \text{...(6)}$$

where $K_1 = \dfrac{L}{A_1E_1}$, $K_2 = \dfrac{L}{A_2E_2}$ and $K_3 = \dfrac{L}{A_3E_3}$

Values of R_1 and R_3 can be obtained from equation (5) and (4) respectively.

Case 2 :

If the support B is not there, beam AC will also deflect due to the load R_2 applied at its centre. Here the total central deflection of point E, relative to its original position, as given by the expression (2) is equal to the elongation of member BE plus the central deflection of beam ABC

$$\frac{R_2L}{A_2E_2} + \frac{R_2L_3}{6EI} = \frac{1}{2}\left(\frac{R_1L}{A_1E_1} + \frac{R_3L}{A_3E_3}\right) + \frac{11}{96} \frac{WL^3}{EI} - \frac{R_2L^3}{6EI} \qquad \text{...(3A)}$$

Solving eqns. (3A) (4) and (5) for R_1, R_2 and R_3 simultaneously.

$$R_2 = \frac{W}{2} \times \frac{3K_1 + K_3 + \dfrac{11}{12} \dfrac{L^3}{EI}}{K_1 + 4K_2 + K_3 + \dfrac{4}{3} \dfrac{L^3}{EI}} \qquad \text{...(7)}$$

In expressions (6) and (7) the quantity K = L/AE for any spring (used as suspension rod here) is the extension of the spring per kg of weight. This may be determined for individual springs.

Procedure :

1. Plot graphs between load applied and tension in each spring. From graph determine the value of stiffness K (extension per unit load) for each spring.
2. Tighten the screw at top for case 1 to make the supports rigid. Load the beam DEF at quarter point and measure extensions of springs. Start with intitial load of 1 kg with increments of 1 kg and maximum load of 4 kg.
3. For case 2, release the middle screws so that the top beam also becomes operative. Load the lower beam at quarter point and measure elongations with initial load of 1 kg with increments of 1 kg and maximum load of 4 kg.

Observations : (A)

S. No.	Spring AD		Spring BE		Spring CF	
	Load	Extension	Load	Extension	Load	Extension
1.	0		0		0	
2.	1 kg		1 kg		1 kg	
3.	2 kg		2 kg		2 kg	
4.	3 kg		3 kg		3 kg	

(B) *Case I*

S. No.	Load	Reading at		
		R_1 (Reaction)	R_2 (Reaction)	R_3 (Reaction)
1.	0			
2.	1 kg			
3.	2 kg			
4.	3 kg			
5.	4 kg			

(C) *Case II*

S. No.	Load	Reading at		
		R_1	R_2	R_3
1.	0			
2.	1 kg			
3.	2 kg			
4.	3 kg			

Calculations : $I = \dfrac{1}{12} bt^3$ for rod ABC and DEF

S. No.	Spring	$K = \left(\dfrac{Load}{Extension}\right)^{-1}$
1.	AD	$K_1 =$
2.	BE	$K_2 =$
3.	CF	$K_3 =$

For Case I :

$$R_2 = \frac{W}{2} \times \frac{3K_1 + K_3 + \dfrac{11}{12}\dfrac{L^3}{EI}}{K_1 + 4K_2 + K_3 + \dfrac{2}{3}\dfrac{L^3}{EI}}$$

$$R_1 = \frac{3}{4} W - \frac{R_2}{2}$$

$$R_1 + R_2 + R_3 = W$$

S. No.	Load	R_1	R_2	R_3
1.	1 kg			
2.	2 kg			
3.	3 kg			
4.	4 kg			

For Case II :

$$R_2 = \frac{3K_1 + K_3 + \dfrac{11}{12}\dfrac{L^3}{EI}}{K_1 + 4K_2 + K_3 + \dfrac{2}{3}\dfrac{L^3}{EI}} \times \frac{W}{2}$$

$$R_1 = \frac{3W}{4} - \frac{R_2}{2}$$

$$R_1 + R_2 + R_3 = W$$

S. No.	Load	R_1	R_2	R_3
1.	1 kg			
2.	2 kg			
3.	3 kg			
4.	4 kg			

Results :

Comparision of results

Applied load		R_1	R_2	R_3
Case I				
1 kg	obs			
	cal			
2 kg	obs			
	cal			
3 kg	obs			
	cal			
Case II				
1 kg	obs			
	cal			
2 kg	obs			
	cal			
3 kg	obs			
	cal			

Object :

To present the experimental study of a three hinged arch for a given system of loading and to compare the results with those obtained analytically.

Apparatus :

Model of a three hinged arch, weight, scale, etc.

Theoretical background :

A three hinged arch is a statically determinate structure. Tthe horizontal thrust for a number of loads is obtained as follows :

Find the reaction V_A and V_B for a simply supported beam AB, which are given as

$$V_A = \frac{1}{L} [W_1 (L - a_1) + W_2 (L - a_2) + W_3 (L - a_3)] \qquad \text{...(1)}$$

$$V_B = \frac{1}{L} (W_1 a_1 + W_3 a_3)$$

$$\sum H = 0; \ H_A + H_B = H$$

$$\sum V = 0; \ V_A + V_B = W_1 + W_2 + W_3$$

To obtain the value of H, take moments about the central hinge C, of all the forces to one side of it. We get

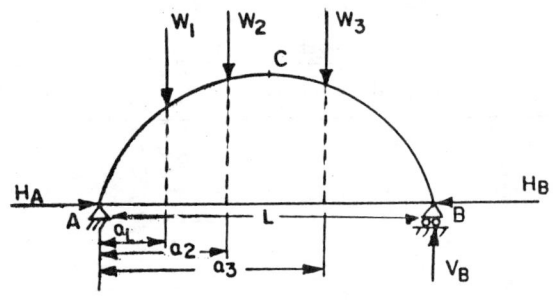

$$H \times h = V_B \times \frac{L}{2} - W_3 \left(a_3 - \frac{L}{2} \right)$$

$$\text{or,} \quad H = \frac{1}{h} \left[V_B \times \frac{L}{2} - W_3 \left(a_3 - \frac{L}{2} \right) \right]$$

Knowing all other quantities, H can be found out.

Procedure :

1. First of all balance the self weight of the arch by putting load on the thrust hanger till the appropriate equilibrium conditions are obtained. Position the movable end of the arch such that it shows a tendency to move inside on tapping the table. Note the load to the nearest 1/4 kg.

2. Place a few loads, two to three in number and in magnitude from 1 to 2 kg on the arch at chosen positions. Once again balance the arch by putting additional weights in the hanger to provide the thrust. The additional weights on the thrust hanger give the experimetnal value of the horizontal thrust.

Observations :

Span of the arch, L =

Central rise, h =

Initial load on thrust hanger to balance self weight of arch =

S. No.	Load applied on hanger	Distance from left hand support	Additional load on thrust hanger, i.e., H
Set 1			
1.	W_1 =	a_1 =	
2.	W_2 =	a_2 =	
3.	W_3 =	a_3 =	
Set 2			
1.	W_4 =	a_4 =	
2.	W_5 =	a_5 =	
3.	W_6 =	a_6 =	

Calculations :

$$V_A = \frac{1}{L} [W_1 (L - a_1) + W_2 (L - a_2) + W_3 (L - a_3)]$$

$$V_B = \frac{1}{L} [W_1 a_1 + W_2 a_2 + W_3 a_3]$$

$$H = \frac{1}{h} \left[V_B \times \frac{1}{2} - W_3 \left(a_3 - \frac{L}{2} \right) \right]$$

S. No.	Observed H	Calculated $H = \frac{1}{2} \left(V_B \times \frac{L}{2} - W_a \left(a_2 - \frac{L}{2} \right) \right)$
Set 1		
Set 2		

Result :

Compare the observed and calculated values of H.

Experiment No. 7

Object :

To determine the elastic displacements of curved members experimentally and verification of the values by analytical methods.

Apparatus :

Model with four curved members, dial guages.

Theory :

To find the elastic displacements of curved members, Castigliano's first theorm will be used which states that "Partial derivative of the total strain energy of a structure with respect to any force acting at a point gives the displacement of the point in the direction of the application of force."

The results obtained for the four curved members shall be as follows :

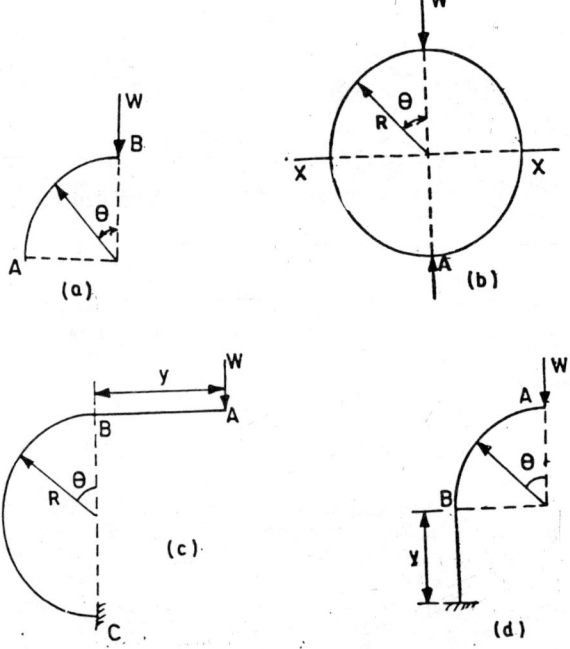

(a) Quadrant of a circle

Fixed at A and free at B and subjected to a concentrated load W at free end.

Vertical displacement of load point, $\Delta BV = \dfrac{\pi WR^3}{4EI}$

Horizontal displacement of load point B, $\Delta BH = \dfrac{WR^3}{2EI}$.

(b) Quadrant with a straight leg

From A to B, quadrant of a circle and from B to C straight.

$$\Delta AV = \frac{\pi WR^3}{4EI} + \frac{WR^2 y}{EI}$$

$$\Delta AH = \frac{WR}{2EI}(R + y)^2$$

(c) Semi circle with straight arm

$$\Delta AV = \frac{Wy^3}{3EI} + \frac{WR}{EI}\left(\pi y^2 + 4yR + \frac{\pi R^2}{2}\right)$$

$$\Delta AH = \frac{WR^2}{EI}(\pi y + 2R)$$

(d) Circle

$$\Delta AV = 0.149\frac{WR^3}{EI}$$

Procedure :

1. Place an initial load 1/2 kg on the hanger. Fix dial guages for horizontal and vertical deflections.
2. Add loads at the ratio of 1/2 kg and tabulate the value of the dial guage readings against the applied loads.
3. In case of a, b and c apply 4 weights each of 1/2 kg. In case of (d) apply 4 weights of 1 kg each.

Results :

Compare the observed and calculated values of displacements.

(a) Quadrant

Load kg	Vert. disp.		Horz. disp.	
	obs.	cal.	obs.	cal.
0				
0.5				
1.0				
1.5				
2.0				

(b) Quadrant with leg

Load kg	Vert. disp.		Horz. disp.	
	obs.	cal.	obs.	cal.
0				
0.5				
1.0				
1.5				
2.0				

(c) Semi-circle with arm

Load kg	Vert. disp.		Horz. disp.	
	obs.	cal.	obs.	cal.
0				
0.5				
1.0				
1.5				
2.0				

(d) Circle

Load kg	Vert. disp.	
	obs.	cal.
0		
1		
2		
3		
4		

Experiment No. 8

Object :

To determine experimentally the horizontal displacement of the roller end of a curved beam due to a given load system and to compare the same with the value obtained theoretically.

Apparatus :

Two hinged arch model, weights, dial gauges.

Theory :

The two hinged arch is a statically indeterminate structure of the first degree. The horizontal thrust is the redundant force. It is determined by strain energy methods. The horizontal outward displacement of the roller end of a curved member due to vertical loads is given by :

$$\int_0^l \frac{M.y.ds}{EI}$$

where

M = bending moment at any point due to loads, as it would be in a simply supported beam

y = rise of the arch axis above base at that point

I = moment of inertia at the point

ds = element length

l = span of the arch.

Take the case of a parabolic arch with a concentrated load W at crown.

$$y = \frac{4h\,x\,(1-x)}{l^2}$$

If $I = I_0 \sec \theta$

where

I_0 = moment of inertia at the crown.

$ds = dx \sec \theta$

$$\int_0^l \frac{M.y.dx}{EI_0} = M = R_A . x$$

$$R_A = R_B = \frac{w}{2}$$

$$M = \frac{W.x}{2} = 2\int_0^{1/2} \frac{W.x}{2EI_0} \times \frac{4hx}{l^2} \times (1-x)\,dx$$

$$= \frac{5}{48}\frac{Wl^2.h}{EI_0}$$

The horizontal movement of the roller end can be found by this method for any position of the load on the arch.

Procedure :

1. Mount a dial gauge to measure the movement of the roller end of the model. Put the lever out of contact.
2. Place a one kg load on hanger at the central position and considering this as the initial loading set the dial gauge to zero reading.
3. Add one kg weight to the hanger and measure the horizontal movement of the roller end.
4. Go on increasing the load (each increment of one kg) till the total is 5 kg and measure the horizontal movement for each increment of load.
5. Unload the hanger (one kg load at a time) and record the horizontal movement of the roller each time.
6. Tabulate load against horizontal movement. Also record values while unloading and compare with the values found theoretically.

Observations and Calculations :

Span of the arch model, l =   Rise of arch =

Central load (kg)		1	2	3	4	5
Observed horizontal movement						
Calculated values of horizontal movement						

Plot a graph between load and horizontal displacement.

Result :

Compare the observed and theoretical values of displacements.

Experiment No. 9

Object :

To obtain experimentally the influence line diagram for horizontal thrust in a three hinged arch and to compare the same with the value obtained theoretically.

Apparatus :

Model of three hinged arch, weights, scale, etc.

Theory :

Influence line is a graph showing the variation of load functions like reactions, bending moments, shear forces, stresses or deflections at a point for varying positions of a unit load on the span.

   Therefore, to draw the influence line for H, we have to place only a load $W = 1$ kg at a varying distance X from other support.

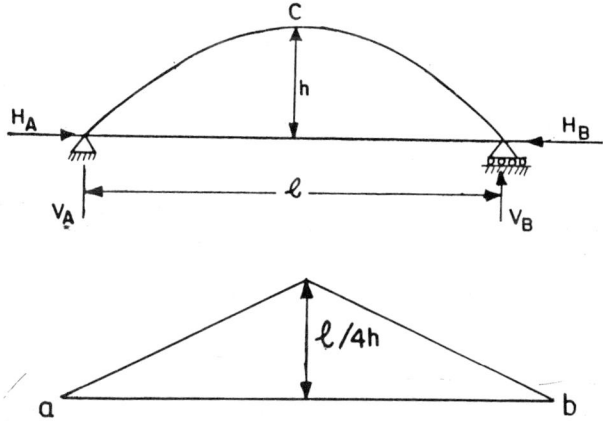

Load between A and C at a distance X from A, considering equilibrium $M_C = 0$

$$1 \times X = V_B \times L$$

$$V_B = \frac{X}{L}$$

$$V_B \times \frac{L}{2} - H_B \times h = 0; \quad H_B = V_B \times \frac{L}{2h}$$

$$H_B = H = 0 \text{ for } X = 0; \quad H_B = \frac{x}{2h}$$

$$H = \frac{L}{4h} \text{ for } X = \frac{L}{2}$$

Load between C and B. Consider a unit load at a distance from A. Considering equilibrium of portion AC, $M_C = 0$

$$V_A \times \frac{L}{2} - H \times h = 0 \quad V_A \times L = 1 \times (L - x)$$

$$H = \frac{L}{4h} \text{ for } X = \frac{L}{2} \quad V_A = L - \frac{x}{L}$$

$$H = 0 \text{ for } X = L \quad H = \frac{V_A}{2Lh}$$

$$H = L - \frac{x}{2h}$$

The influence line for H is shown in the figure.

Procedure :

1. Balance the self weight of the arch by placing the load on the hanger until the equilibrium conditions are obtained.
2. Put a load of 2 kg in turn on each hanger and find the balancing weights required on the thrust hanger for thrust.
3. Plot ordinates representing ½ of the balance weights on the load position as base. This gives the influence line for H.

Observations and Calculations :

Initial load on thrust hanger to balance self weight of arch =

2 kg at hanger No.	1	2	3	4	5	6	7
Balancing weights on thrust hanger (kg)							
Net weights							
Influence line ordinate (observed)							
Influence line ordinate (calculated)							

Result :

Plot two graphs for influence line (observed and calculated values) on the same graph and comment on the accuracy obtained in the above two cases.

Reference for Structural Engineering Laboratory

1. Chameeki, Samuel, Influence Lines for Plane and Three Dimensional Continuous Structures, Paragon Press, London, 4th edition, 1974.
2. Dayarathnam, Pasala; Analysis of Statically Determinate Structures, Affiliated East-West Press, New Delhi, 1st edition, 1976.
3. Jay, B.E., Beam and Frame Analysis, Arnold Press, London, 3rd edition, 1966.
4. Junrarkar, S.B., Mechanics of Structures, Vivek Publishers, Bombay, 3rd edition, 1977.
5. Punmia, B.C. , Strength of Material and Mechanics of Structures, Standard Publishers, New Delhi, 7th edition, 1986.
6. Ramamurtham S., Theory of Structures, Dhanpat Rai and Sons, New Delhi, 2nd edition, 1973.
7. Reddy, C.S., Basic Structural Analysis (in SI units), Tata McGraw Hill Publishing Co. Ltd., New Delhi, 4th edition, 1986.
8. Vazirani V.N. and Ratwani M.M, Analysis Design and Details of Structures, Khanna Publishers, New Delhi, 3rd edition, 1981.

SECTION 7

PUBLIC HEALTH ENGINEERING
LABORATORY

Experiment No. 1

Object

Determination of colour.

Theory :

Many surface waters, particularly those emanating from swampy areas are often coloured to the extent that they are not acceptable for domestic or some industrial uses without treatment to remove the colour. The colouring material results from contact of the water with organic debris, such as leaves, needles of conifers and wood, and various stages of decomposition. It consists of vegetable extracts of a considerable variety. Tannis, humic acids and humates from the decomposition of lagnin, are considered to be the principal colour bodies. Iron is sometimes present as ferric humate and produces a colour of high potency.

Surface waters may appear highly coloured, because of coloured suspended matter, while in reality they are not. In water analysis it is necessary to differentiate this from true colour. Surface-water may become coloured by pollution with highly coloured waste waters from dying operations, textile industries, etc., which are readily recognized and treated.

Waters containing colouring matter derived from natural substances undergoing decay in swamps and forests are not considered to possess harmful or toxic properties. The natural colouring materials, however, give a yellow-brownish appearance to the water, somewhat like that of urine, and there is a natural reluctance on the part of water consumers to drink such waters because of the associations involved. It is this required supply water that is not only hygienically safe but aesthetically acceptable, otherwise consumers are likely to be drawn to waters that may be aesthetically good but of poor hygienic quality. The U.S.P.H. Service recommends that waters intended for human use should not have a colour exceeding 20 units.

The instrument used is Heilige Water Colour and Turbidity Testing Apparatus (U.S.G.S. Model).

Determination of colour of water is done comparing a water sample with one glass colour standard or a combination of two or three standards. One colour unit is equivalent to the colour of a solution containing 1 mg of platinum per liter when viewed in a depth of 200 mm. Thus, a standard with the value 40 has the same colour as a standard solution containing 40 parts of platinum particles per million (ppm). A combination of standards is equal to the sum of the individual standards so that, for example, the standards 20 and 5 together have the same colour as a standard solution containing 25 parts of platinum per million. The value of the standards are so provided that any value between 5 and 145 ppm at intervals of 5 can be obtained by a combination of individual glasses.

Procedure :

Place a water sample in the 200 mm tube if it is moderately coloured. To remove dust or lint, rinse the tube once or twice immediately before use with a portion of the water sample. Fill the 'standard' tube (the tube with the spring clip) with distilled water. If distilled water is not available, use the tube empty.

Make the colour comparison by looking with one eye simultaneously through both tubes. To accomplish this, hold the tubes at a slight angle to each other and with the rear of each tube about 9 inches from the eye so that the sides of the tubes are quite visible.

On a bright day, make the comparison against a white surface such as piece of paper, or tile on which the light falls. On a gray day match the colours by viewing against the sky near the horizon. Good results cannot be obtained by viewing directly against sunlight or artificial light.

Change the colour standard or combination of standards till the colours in the two tubes match. The sum of the numbers on colour standards gives the colour value of the sample. If the colour of the water sample is intermediate between two standards or two combinations of standards, the true result is estimated by interpolation.

Highly Coloured Waters :

When difficulties are encountered in matching water of a colour higher than 70 units, follow either procedure 1 or 2 below.

1. Use the 100 mm tube and multiply the result by 2 or use the 50mm tube and multiply the result by 4. This multiplication is necessary as the glass colour standards represent the indicated values only when compared with a sample in the tube of 200 mm viewing depth.

2. Use the 200 mm tube, dilute the sample with distilled water, and multiply the reading by the dilution factor. For example, if one volume of sample is diluted with the same volume of distilled water, the result must be multiplied by 2. If one volume of sample is diluted with three volumes of distilled water, the result must be multiplied by 4, etc. For measuring the sample and distilled water the tube itself may be used.

Interference of Turbidity :

Slight turbidity will not interfere with colour determinations. If the water sample shows a pronounced turbidity it should be filtered through a heavy filter power. However, since filters exert marked decolorizing action, the removal of the ended matter is best done by centrifuging the sample before making the colour determination.

Precautions :

Cleanliness is of utmost importance in all colour determinations. Dirt of any kind, even figure marks on the glass colour standards, or cover glasses of the tubes, may cause in-accurate results. Hence perform the experiment with the clearest possible way.

Do not allow the water to dry out in the tubes. Always wash and dry tubes and cover glasses immediately after use and stack them in the case protected from dust and damage.

Experiment No. 2

Object :

Determination of turbidity.

Theory :

The term turbid is applied to waters containing suspended matter that interferes with the passage of light through the water. The turbidity may be caused by a wide variety of suspended material, which range in size from colloidal to coarse dispersions, depending upon the degree of turbulence. In rivers under flood conditions, turbidity will be due to relatively coarse dispersions.

Turbidity is an important consideration in public water supplies. Turbid waters are objected to by consumers because of their appearance and because of their possible association with sewage pollution and health hazard occassioned by it. Filteration of water is rendered more difficult and costly when turbidity increases. Turbidity may also affect the efficiency of disinfection.

An arbitrary standard has been adopted to express turbidity. The standard is 1 mg of SiO_2/litre = 1 unit of turbidity and the silica used must meet certain specifications.

The U.S.P.H. Service has placed a limit of 10 units of turbidity as the maximum amount allowable in public water supplies.

Instruments and Procedures :

Paterson turbidity meter and Hellige turbidity testing apparatus are described below :

1. *Paterson Turbidity Meter :* The Paterson turbidity meter is an optical instrument designed to enable the clarify of water or other liquids with ease and rapidity, and at the same time to ensure that such determination is accurate and comparable to recognised standard.

Briefly described, the apparatus consists of a vertical ebonite body which has been specially designed to hold one litre of water (although the quantity is not important provided the mirrors are completely covered). On the back and front faces of the body, protected by aluminium back plates, are mounted two mirrors (the reflecting surfaces of which face each other at a slight predetermined angle). In each mirror an aperture is formed, one of these permitting the passage of a light ray from a lamp of standard strength, whilst the other allows the opposing mirror to be viewed. The ebonite head contains the mechanism by which a slider can be raised or lowered, and is removable for filling and/or cleaning purposes. This slider is actuated by the ebonite knob on the right hand side of the head.

On filling the instrument and switching on the attached electric light, multiple reflections are obtained of the original light spot. These reflections being visible as a row of light spots. Visibility is being a measure of the turbidity of the fluid under examination.

2. *Hellige Apparatus :* For turbidity measurement, it consists of a graduated and marked tape at the end of which is attached a graduated aluminium strip, and a platinum needle.

Following procedure is used to determine turbidity.

1.   Insert the screw-eye into the aluminium strip so that the platinum needle projects from the side with the scale.

2. Insert the end of a 3 ft long stick into the opening of the screw-eye. Hold the tape taut, immerse the aluminium strip in the water, and observe the needle from the point marked "PLACE EYE HERE" at the upper end of the tape.

3. When the needle just disappears read the depth of immersion from the scale on the tape. The number indicates the turbidity directly in parts per million (ppm) of suspended silica.

4. If the water is so turbid that the Needle disappears when the aluminium strip is immersed, take the reading from the scale of the latter.

Precautions :

1. Measurement must always be made in the open, preferably during the middle of the day. If the sun is shining, the observer should take such a position that this shadow covers the water around the stick and needle.

2. If the water is agitated by waves or currents, if the depth of the water is not sufficient to immerse the strip until the needle disappears, or if for any other reason the measurement cannot be made properly, a pail or tub may be filled with the water and the reading should be taken immediately before any particles have settled.

3. For highest accuracy the diameter of the vessel must be at least twice the depth to which the needle is immersed.

4. Dry all parts of the apparatus before they are replaced in the case.

Experiment No. 3

Object :

Determination of the pH value of water.

Theory :

pH is the logarithm of the reciprocal of the hydrogen ion concentration — more precisely, of hydrogen ion activying — in moles per litre. The practical pH scale extends from 0 (very acidic), to 14 (very alkaline), with middle value corresponding to exact neutrality at 25°C. Whereas, alkalinity and acidity express the total reserve or buffering capacity of a sample, the pH value represents the instantaneous hydrogen ion activity.

pH enters into calculation of carbonate, bicarbonate, and carbon dioxide, as well as of the corrosion or stability index and into the control of water and waste water treatment processes.

The pH of most natural waters falls within the range of 4 to 9. The majority of waters are slightly basic due to the presence of carbonate and bicarbonate. A departure from the normal for a given water could be caused by the entry of strongly acidic or basic industrial wastes. A relatively common practice is the pH adjustment of treatment plant effluent for the purpose of controlling corrosion in the distribution system.

Methods of pH measurement :

pH can be measured by two methods, colorimetrically and electrometrically. The colorimetric methods suffer from severe interference contributed by colour, turbidity, high saline content, celloidal matter, free chlorine, and various oxidants and reductants. The indicators are subjected to deterioration, as are and colour standards with which they are compared. Moreover no single indicator encompasses the pH range of interest in water. For these reasons, the colorimetric method is suitable only for rough estimation and is not considered good for the detailed determination of pH value. The electrometric method also known as Glass Electrode Method is considered standard.

Glass Electrode Method : This method involves use of an equipment called pH meter, with a pair of electrodes. Several types of electrodes have been suggested for electrometric determination of pH. Although the hydrogen gas electrode is recognized as the primary standard, the glass electrode ion combination with the reference potential provided by a saturated calomel electrode is most generally used.

When a pair of electrodes namely pH sensitive glass electrode and a reference electrode are dipped in an aqueous solution, they generate e.m.f. which is proportional to the pH of the solution (change of 1 pH unit produces an electrical charge of 59.1 mV at 25°C. The pH meter essentially measures this electrical change and gives direct reading of pH over a calibrated scale. Necessary feedbacks are incorporated to achieve good stability and freedom from aging compensation for temperature and asymmetry potential effect is also incorporated in the instrument.

In our laboratory we have SYSTRONICS pH meter Type 322. For specifications and other details and manual available in the laboratory may be consulted. The procedure described below for determination of pH value is as prescribed by the manufacturer.

Procedure :

1. Keep the CHECK/ZERO/READ switch in ZERO position. Switch on the instrument. After one minute,

adjust the zero by 'SET ZERO' control. Then allow ten minutes for warming and to stabilize. Wash the electrodes by a jet of distilled water and wipe them with a soft tissue paper or filter paper.

2.   Immerse the electrodes in the beaker containing standard buffer solution. Set 'RANGE' switch in appropriate pH range. Set the zero (7 pH) by 'SET ZERO' control, accurately making use of the mirror on the scale. Measure temperature in degrees centigrade of the solution by a thermometer and set this value on the 'TEMPCOM' control. Then set the CHECK/ZERO/READ switch in the READ position. Now set the buffer pH value on the meter by means of 'CALIBRATE' control. Put back the ZERO/READ switch in ZERO position. Now the meter is standardized. Take out the electrodes. Wash them with distilled water and wipe them with filter paper.

3.   To measure the pH of unknown solution, immerse the electrodes in that solution, select the proper range in the 'RANGE' switch. Set the ZERO/READ switch in 'READ' position and read the pH indicated by the meter on the scale to which 'RANGE' is set. The scale reads pH 7-14 from left to right and pH 0-7 from right to left.

4.   When a series of measurements are being taken, check the zero and correct it, if necessary, by putting ZERO/READ switch in 'ZERO' position and then adjusting 'SET ZERO' control.

Result :

The pH value of water =

Standard (recommended value) =

The recommended value of pH =

Experiment No. 4

Object :

Determination of acidity.

Theory :

The acidity of a water is the capacity of the water to donate protons. This includes the un-ionized portions of weakly ionizing acids such as carbonic acid and tannic acid, as well as hydrolyzing salts like ferrous and/or aluminium sulfate. Mineral acids contribute to acidity when the sample has a low pH value. The acidity is significant because acids contribute to the corrosiveness of water.

Acidity is expressed as equivalent quantity of $CaCO_3$ in mg/litre.

Principle : An equilibrium between carbonate, bicarbonate, and carbon dioxide exists in many natural waters used for potable purposes. The carbonate and bicarbonate can be estimated by titrating the alkalinity with standard acid to bicarbonate equivalence point of pH 8.3 and then to the carbonic acid equivalence point in the pH range of ·4 to 5. Acid pollutant entering a water supply in sufficient quantity will disturb the carbonate-bicarbonate-carbon dioxide equilibrium. The extent of this disturbance may be estimated by titrating with standard alkali to the end points of pH 4.5 and 8.3.

The titration of the sample at boiling temperature in the presence of phenolphthalein indicator has been found useful for water plant control where the source of supply is polluted with mineral acids and acid salts originating from acid in the drainage and some industrial wastes. Heat speeds up the hydrolysis of iron and aluminium sulfate, enabling rapid completion of the titration. This provides an estimate of the lime application which may be required to make such water supplies satisfactory for general use.

Apparatus : Burette, Erlenmeyer flask.

Reagents : Phenolphthalein indicator solution, standard sodium hydroxide titrant, 0.02 N.

Procedure

1. Take 25 ml of sample. Remove the free available residual chlorine from the sample by adding 0.05 ml (1 drop), 0.1 sodium thiosulfate solution.
2. Add 0.15-0.5 ml (3-10 drops) phenolphthalein indicator to a sample of suitable size, 50 to 100 ml, if possible, in an Erlenmeyer flask.
3. Heat the sample for 2 minutes.
4. Titrate the hot sample with standard 0.02 N NaOH to a permanent pink end point.

Calculations :

$$\text{Acidity as mg/l } CaCO_3 = \frac{A \times N \times 50000}{\text{ml of sample}}$$

where

    A = ml of NaOH

    N = normality of NaOH

Experiment No. 5

Object :

Determination of alkalinity.

Theory :

The alkalinity of water is the capacity of water to accept protons. It is a measure of the basic constituents of water. Alkalinity is usually imparted by bicarbonate, normal carbonate and hydroxide components of a natural or treated water.

Within reasonable limits alkalinity has no sanitary significance, but it is very important in connection with coagulation, softening and corrosion prevention. Alum is an acid salt which, when added in small quantities to natural water, reacts with the alkalinity present to form floc. If insufficient alkalinity is present to react with all the alum, coagulation will be incomplete and soluble alum will be left in water. It may, therefore, be necessary to add alkalinity in the form of soda ash or lime to complete the coagulation or to maintain sufficient alkalinity to prevent the coagulated water from being corrosive. Alkalinity is expressed as equivalent quantity of $CaCO_3$ in mg/litre.

Principle :

Total alkalinity can be determined by titration with a standard solution of a strong mineral acid using methyl orange indicator. In order to distinguish between the kinds of alkalinity present in a sample and to determine the quantity of each, titration is made using two indicators — phenolphthalein and methyl orange — successfully.

Phenolphthalein gives pink colour only in the presence of hydroxide or normal carbonate. The change from pink to colourless occurs at pH value of 8.3. Methyl orange is yellow in presence of any of the three types of alkalinity and red in the presence of acid. The change in colour occurs at a pH value of approximately 4.4.

Normal carbonate alkalinity may be present with either hydroxide or bicarbonate alkalinity, but hydroxide and bicarbonate cannot be present together in the same sample. If there is phenolphthalein alkalinity in a sample, it is due to the presence of either hydroxide or normal carbonate or both. If there is methyl orange alkalinity present, it is due to any one of the three alkalinities or hydroxide and normal carbonate together or normal carbonate and bicarbonate together.

The following equations illustrate the reactions occuring when each of the three types of alkalinity is titrated with an acid :

1. Hydroxide :

   $2NaOH + H_2SO_4 = Na_2SO_4 + 2H_2O$

2. Normal carbonate :

   $2Na_2CO_3 + H_2SO_4 = 2NaHCO_3 + Na_2SO_4$

   $2NaHCO + H_2SO_4 = Na_2SO_4 + 2H_2CO_3$

3. Bicarbonate :

   $2NaHCO_3 + H_2SO_4 = Na_2SO_4 + 2H_2CO_3$

It may be noted that when normal carbonate is present in the phenolphthalein, end point will be reached when half of the normal carbonate reaction is completed. The other half of the reaction would be completed in the methyl orange range. This fact is made use of in developing interrelationship among total alkalinity, alkalinity indicated by phenolphthalein and alkalinity indicated by methyl orange which help in determining the quantities of different types of alkalinities as shown in the following table.

Following five alkalinity conditions are possible in a sample :

(1) Hydroxide alone, (2) Hydroxide and normal carbonate, (3) Normal carbonate alone, (4) Normal carbonate and bicarbonate, and (5) Bicarbonate alone.

Table : Alkalinity Relationships

Result of titration	Hydroxide Alkalinity as CaCO₃	Carbonate Alkalinity as CaCO₃	Bicarbonate Alkalinity as CaCO₃
$P = 0$	0	0	T
$P < 1/2T$	0	2P	T – 2P
$P = 1/2T$	0	2P	0
$P > 1/2T$	2P – T	2 (T – P)	0
$P = T$	T	0	0

where

P = phenolphthalein alkalinity

T = total alkalinity = phenolphthalein alkalinity + methyl orange alkalinity when successive titration of the same sample is done first using phenolphthalein indicator and then methyl orange indicator.

Apparatus :

Burette, Erlenmeyer flask

Reagents :

Carbon oxide free distilled water, phenolphthalein indicator solution, methyl orange indicator solution, standard sulfuric acid solution (0.02 N).

Procedure :

1. Take 25 ml of sample. Remove the free residual chlorine from the water sample by adding 0.05 ml (1 drop) 0.1 N sodium thiosulfate solution.
2. Add 0.1 ml (2 drops) phenolphthalein indicator to a sample of suitable size if no change in colour, phenolphthalein alkaline is absent and proceed to step No. 4.
3. If the colour of sample changes to pink on addition of phenolphthalein indicator, titrate it over a white surface with 0.02 N standard sulfuric acid solution till it is colourless. Note the ml of the acid solution consumed.
4. Add 0.15 ml (3 drops) methyl orange indicator to the same sample. Titrate over a white surface with 0.02 N standard sulfuric acid solution till the colour changes from yellow to red. Note the ml of the acid solution consumed.

Calculations :

(i) Phenolphthalein alkalinity as mg/l $CaCO_3$ = $\dfrac{P \times N \times 50000}{\text{ml sample}}$

(ii) Total alkaiinity as mg/l $CaCO_3$ = $\dfrac{T \times N \times 50000}{\text{ml sample}}$

(iii) Methyl alkalinity = (ii) − (i)

where

P = ml of titrant for sample to reach the phenolphthalein end point

   = P + ml of titrant for sample to reach the methyl orange end point

N = Normality of standard acid solution.

Experiment No. 6

Object :

To determine the hardness.

Theory :

Water is universal solvent and dissolves varying amounts of different mineral substances. Those producing hardness do not affect the sanitary quality but are of importance in the domestic use of water, particularly for laundry and boiler purposes. Calcium and magnesium salts, the principal mineral constituents, consume soap and precipitate as insoluble compounds or soap curds until all the calcium and magnesium is precipitated, no lather or washing action is obtained from the soap; the soap consuming power of water is, therefore, a measure of its hardness. Calcium and magnesium generally are dissolved as soluble bicarbonate but may change, owing to heating, to the less soluble carbonate which precipitates and is one source of scale in distributing systems and hot-water heaters. Hard waters are usually less corrosive than soft waters.

Principle (EDTA Method) : Ethylene diaminetetra-acetic acid and its sodium salts (abbreviated EDTA) form a chelated soluble complex when added to a solution of certain metal cations. If a small amount of a dye such as chrome black T is added to an aqueous solution containing calcium and magnesium ions at a pH of 10.0 + 0.1 the solution will become wine red. If EDTA is then added as titrant, the calcium and magnesium will be complexed. After sufficient EDTA has been added to complex, the solution will turn from wine red to blue. This is the end point of the titration. The sharpness of the end point increases with increasing pH, however, cannot be increased indefinitely because of the danger of precipitating $CaCO_3$ or $Mg(OH)_2$, and because the dye changes colour at high pH values. The pH value of 10.0 + 0.1 (recommended in this procedure) is a satisfactory compromise. A limit (5 min) is set for the duration of the titration in order to minimise the tendency towards $CaCO_3$ precipitation.

Some metal ions interfere with this procedure by causing fading or indistinct end points. This interference is reduced by the addition of certain inhibitors to the water sample prior to titration with EDTA.

Apparatus : Burette.

Reagents : Buffer solution, chrome black T indicator, standard EDTA titrant, 0.01 N (1 ml = 1.000 mg $CaCO_3$)

Procedure :

1. Dilute 25 ml of sample to about 50 ml with distilled water in suitable vessel.
2. Add 1-2 ml of buffer solution to give a pH value of 10.0 to 10.1.
3. Add 1-2 drops of indicator solution.
4. Add the standard EDTA slowly with continuous stirring, until the last reddish tinge disappears from the solution, adding the last few drops at 3-5 seconds intervals. The colour of the solution at the end point is blue under normal conditions.

Calculations :

$$\text{Hardness (EDTA) as mg/l } CaCO_3 = \frac{\text{ml EDTA titrant} \times 1000 \times f}{\text{ml sample}}$$

where $f = \dfrac{\text{mg } CaCO_3}{\text{ml EDTA titrant}}$

Experiment No. 7

Object :

To determine the calcium in water.

Theory :

The presence of calcium in water results from passage through or over deposits of limestone, dolomite, gypsum, and gypsiferous scale. The calcium content may range from zero to several hundred mg/l, depending on the source and treatment of water. Small concentrations of calcium carbonate combat corrosion of metallic pipes by laying down a protective coating. Appropriate calcium salts, on the other hand, breakdown on heating to form harmful scales in boilers, pipes and cooking utensils. Calcium content of water is one of the important variables in the theoretical and practical studies of the scale formation and corrosive properties of water.

Chemical softening treatment or ion exchange is employed to reduce the calcium and the associated hardness to tolerable levels.

Principle (EDTA Titrimetric Method)

When EDTA (ethylene diaminetetra acetic acid) or its salt is added to water containing both calcium and magnesium, it combines first with calcium that is present. Calcium can be determined directly using EDTA. When the pH is made sufficiently high that the magnesium is largely precipitated as the hydroxide and an indicator is used which combines with calcium only. Several indicators are available that will give a colour change at the point where all the calcium has been complexed by EDTA at a pH of 12-13.

Apparatus :

Pipette, burette, Erlenmeyer flask, etc.

Reagents :

Sodium hydroxide (1 N), murexide (ammonium purpurate) indicator, standard EDTA titrant (0.01 N).

Procedure :

(*Note :* Because of high pH used in this procedure, perform the titration immediately after addition of the alkali).

1. Take 50 ml of sample so that the calcium content is about 5-10 mg in an Erlenmeyer flask. Analyze hardwater with alkalinity higher than 300 mg/l $CaCO_3$ by taking a smaller amount of sample diluting it to 50 ml, or by neutralizing the alkalinity with acid, boiling for 1 minute and cooling before beginning the titration.

2. Add 2.0 ml NaOH solution, or a volume sufficient to produce a pH of 12-13. Stir.

3. Add 0.1-0.2 g of the murexide indicator (or drops if a solution is used).

4. Add EDTA titrant slowly with continuous stirring to the proper end point. Murexide indicator changes from pink to purple at the end point by adding 1-2 drops of titrant in excess to make certain that no further colour change occurs.

Calculations :

(i) mg/l Ca $= \dfrac{A \times B \times 400.8}{\text{ml sample}}$

(ii) Calcium hardness as mg/l $CaCO_3 = \dfrac{A \times B \times 1000}{\text{ml sample}}$

where

A = ml titration for sample, and

B = mg $CaCO_3$ equivalent to 1.00 ml of EDTA titrant at the calcium indicator end point.

Experiment No. 8

Object :

To determine the chlorides in water.

Theory :

The test for the content of chloride in water may be used for various purposes :

1. Salt is present in sewage from urine in the range of about 50-200 mg/l and higher yet in countries with low water consumption per capita, so the content of chlorides in polluted water is a rough measure of the degree of solution. This is especially the case with well waters, in which seepage from cess-pools in the ground water tributary of a well may be disclosed. This, however, required that the normal chloride content of the unpolluted surface and ground waters be known for comparison purposes. For instance, the normal content in ground water in a given neighbourhood may be 0.5 mg/l, so a content of, say, 2.2 mg/l in a well water in the vicinity would disclose significant seepage.

2. Water has salty taste to some people when the contents of chlorides exceeds about 150 mg/l and 200 mg/l is the maximum desirable contents. A high chloride content also exerts a deleterious effect on metallic pipes and structures, as well as on agricultural plants.

3. The chloride content of ground waters is used in the study of salt-water intrusion along the sea coast, which destroys the usefulness of wells so affected. Local deposits of rock salt naturally lead to high chloride content in ground waters — that is salty water not related to pollution or sea water intrusion — and hence without sanitary signification.

4. The test for chloride is used in the control of the regeneration of ion-exchange software with solutions of salt.

Principle :

In a neutral or slightly alkaline solution, potassium chromate can be used to indicate the end point of the silver nitrate titration of chloride. Silver chloride is quantitatively precipitated before red silver chromate is formed.

Substances in amounts normally found in potable waters will not interfere. However, the sample may have to be pretreated for eliminating interference.

Equations :

$$NaCl + AgNO_3 = AgCl + NaNO_3$$
(white precipitate)

$$2AgNO_3 + K_2CrO_4 = Ag_2CrO_4 + 2KNO_3$$

Apparatus :

Burette, 1 ml pipette.

Reagents :

Potassium chromate indicator solution, standard silver nitrate titrant (0.0141 N).

Procedure :

1. Take 100 ml of sample or a suitable aliquot diluted to 100 ml in Erlenmeyer flask. Take 100 ml of distilled water in another Erlenmeyer flask.
2. Adjust the pH of the sample in the range 7-10 with sulfuric acid or sodium hydroxide solution.
3. Add 1 ml of potassium chromate K_2CrO_4 indicator solution to each flask.
4. Titrate the sample with standard silver nitrate titrant to a pinkish yellow end point.
5. Establish the reagent black value by the titration method outlined above. A blend of 0.2 to 0.3 ml is usual for the method.

Calculations :

$$\text{mg/l Cl} = \frac{(A - B) \times N \times 35450}{\text{ml of sample}}$$

where

A = ml of titrant for sample

B = ml of titrant for blank

N = normality of $AgNO_3$.

Experiment No. 9

Object :

To determine the fluorides in water.

Theory :

Fluorides occur naturally in many public water supplies and, if present in drinking water in excess of 1.0-1.5 mg of fluoride per litre, they may give rise to dental fluorosis in some children. When present in much higher concentrations, they may eventually, cause endemic cumulative fluorosis with resultant skeletal damage in both children and adults.

In assessing the safety of water supply with respect to the above limits of fluoride concentration, special consideration could be given to the total daily fluoride intake by the individual. Apart from variations in climatic conditions, it is well known that in some areas certain food substances contain fluorides; consequently, due attention should be given to both these factors. It should be emphasized, therefore, that in those areas where fluoride containing foods are ingested, the lower limit of the above concentration range should be guiding factor as to the chemical quality of the water.

Fluoride is also regarded as an essential constituent of drinking water, particularly with regard to the prevention of dental caries in children. If the fluoride concentration in the drinking water of a community is less than 0.5 mg/l, a high incidence of dental caries is likely to occur. To prevent the development of dental caries in children, a number of communal water supplies are fluoridated to bring the fluoride concentration to 1.0 mg/l.

Accurate determination of fluoride in water is, therefore, important in maintaining the effectiveness and safety of the fluoridation procedure.

Principle : (Alizatin Visula Method)

Among the many methods suggested for the determination of fluoride ion in water, the electrode and colorimetric methods are believed to be the most satisfactory at the present time. They are based on the reaction between fluoride and a zirconium-dye lake. The fluoride reacts with the dye lake, dissociating a portion of it into colourless complex ion (ZF^{2-}) and the dye. As the amount of fluoride is increased, the colour produced becomes progressively lighter different in hue, depending on the reagent used.

Because all of the methods are subject to errors where interfering ions are present, it may be necessary to distill the sample prior to making the fluoride determination. When interfering ions are not present in excess of the tolerances of the method, the fluoride determination may be made directly without distillation.

Apparatus :

Nessler tubes, pipette.

Reagents :

Standard sodium fluoride solution (1 ml = 100 µg of fluoride); acid-zirconyl-alizarin reagent.

Procedure :

1. Take 50 ml of sample. If the sample contains residual chlorine, remove it by adding 1 drop (0.05 ml) of sodium arsenite solution for each 0.1 mg. of chlorine and mix.
2. Prepare a series of standards by diluting various volumes of standard fluoride solution to 100 ml in Nessler tubes.
3. Adjust the temperature of samples and standards so that the deviation between them is no more than 2°C.
4. To 100 ml of clear sample and the standards in Nessler tubes, add 5 ml of the acid-Zircony reagent from a volumetric pipette. Mix thoroughly taking care to avoid contamination during the process.
5. After each 1 μg, compare the sample with standards and note the μg of fluoride in the matching standard.

Calculations :

$$\text{mg/l fluoride} = \frac{A}{\text{ml sample}} \times \frac{B}{C}$$

where

A = μg fluoride in matched standard.

The ratio B/C applies only when a sample is diluted to volume B.

Experiment No. 10

Object :

To find out the dissolved oxygen in water.

Theory :

Adequate dissolved oxygen (DO) is necessary for the life of fish and other aquatic organisms. The DO concentration may also be associated with corrosivity of water, photosynthetic activity and septicity. The DO test is used in biochemical oxygen demand (BOD) determination as carried out by the dilution method.

In the determination of DO, there are various ions and compounds which cause interference. To correct for these interferences, numerous modifications of the basic Winkler method have been proposed. The choice of the exact procedure to be used will depend upon the nature of the sample and the interferences present. The Alsterberg (sodium oxide) modification which is used for most sewage, effluents, and streams especially if they contain more than 0.1 mg/l nitrite and not more than 1 mg/l ferrous. Other reducing or oxidizing materials should be absent. If 1 ml potassium fluoride solution is added before acidifying the sample and there is no delay in titration, the method is also applicable in the presence of 100-200 mg/l of ferric.

Principle :

The basic Winkler procedure entails the oxidation of manganous hydroxide in a highly alkaline solution. Upon acidification in the presence of an iodide, the manganic hydroxide dissolves and free iodine is liberated in an amount equivalent to the oxygen originally dissolved in the sample the free iodine is titrated with a sodium thiosulfate standard solution, using starch as an internal indicator, after most of the iodine has been reduced. The normality of the thiosulfate solution is adjusted so that 1 ml is equivalent to 1 mg/l dissolved oxygen when 200 ml of the original sample is titrated.

Sampling :

Collect the sample in narrow-mouth, glass-stoppered bottles of 250-300 ml capacity. Special precautions are required to avoid entrainment or solution of atmospheric oxygen. In sampling, a glass or rubber tube attached to the tap should extend to the bottom of the bottle. Allow the bottle to overflow two or three times its volume and replace the stopper, so that no air bubbles are entrained. The temperature of the sampled water should be recorded to the nearest degree centigrade.

There should be no delay in the determination of DO on all samples that contain an appreciable iodine demand. If the Alsterberg modification is to be used, preservation of samples for 4-8 hrs is accomplished by adding 0.7 ml conc. H_2SO_4 and 1 ml sodium azide (2 g NaN_3 ub 100 ml distilled water) to the DO bottle. This will arrest biologic activity and maintain the DO if the bottle is stored at the temperature of collection or water sealed and kept at a temperature of 10-20°C.

Reagents :

Manganous sulfate solution, alkali-iodine-azide reagent, conc. sulfuric acid, starch solution, sodium thiosulfate stock solution (0.10 N), standard sodium thiosulfate solution (0.02 N), potassium fluoride solution.

Procedure :

To the sample as collected in a 250-300 ml bottle, add 2 ml $MnSO_4$ solution followed by 2 ml alkali-iodide-azide reagent, well below the surface of the liquid stopper with care to exclude air bubbles and mix by inverting the bottle several times. When the precipitate settles, leaving a clear supernatent above the manganese hydroxide floc, shake again. When setting has produced at least 100 ml clear supernatent carefully remove the stopper and immediately add 2.0 ml conc. H_2SO_4 by allowing the acid to run down the neck of the bottle, and mix by gentle inversion until dissolution is complete. The iodine should be uniformly distributed throughout the bottle before decanting the amount needed for titration. This should correspond to 200 ml of the original sample after correction for the loss corresponds to 200 ml of the original sample after correction for the loss of sample by displacement with the reagents has been made. Thus, when a total of 4 ml (2 ml each) of the manganous sulfate and alkali-iodide-azide reagents is added to a 300-ml bottle, the volume taken for titration should be

$$200 \times \frac{300}{300-4} = 203 \text{ ml.}$$

Titrate with 0.025 N thiosulfate to a pale straw colour.

Add 1-2 ml freshly prepared starch solution and continue the titration the first disappearance of the blue colour. Subsequent recolorations due to the catalytic effect of nitrite or to traces of ferric salts which have not been complexed with fluoride should be disregarded.

Calculations :

Since 1 ml 0.02 N $Na_2S_2O_3$ is equivalent to 0.2 mg DO, each milliliter of sodium thiosulfate used is equivalent to 1 mg/l DO if a volume equal to 200 ml of original sample is titrated.

If the results are desired in milliliters of oxygen gas per liter at 0°C and 760 mm pressure, multiply mg/l DO by 0.698.

To express the results as per cent saturation at 760 mm atmospheric pressure, the solubility data may be used. Formulae are available for correcting the solubilities to barometric pressures other than mean sea level.

The solubility of DO in distilled water at any barometric pressure, P (mm Hg), temperature, t (degree C), and saturated vapor pressure, u (mm Hg), for the given t, may be calculated between the temperature of 0 and 30°C by Eq. 1, and between 30 and 50°C by Eq. 2 :

$$\text{ml/l DO} = \frac{(P-u) \times 0.678}{35+t} \qquad \qquad ...(1)$$

$$\text{ml/l DO} = \frac{(P-u) \times 0.827}{49+t} \qquad \qquad ...(2)$$

Experiment No. 11

Purpose :

Determination of bio-oxygen demand.

Theory :

The Biochemical Oxygen Demand (BOD) of sewage or polluted water is the amount of oxygen, required for the biological decomposition of dissolved organic matter to occur under aerobic conditions and at a standardized time and temperature. BOD test is among the most important made in sanitary analysis and is used as a generalized measure for the amount of oxidizable matter contained in water or pollutional load placed upon it, as a means of predicting the progress of aerobic decomposition in polluted water and the degree of self-purification accomplished in given interval of time.

The oxygen demand of sewage, sewage plant effluents, polluted waters or industrial wastes is exerted by three classes of materials: (a) Carbonaceous organic material usable as a source of food by aerobic organisms; (b) oxidizable nitrogen derived from nitrite, ammonia and organic nitrogen reducing compounds which will react with molecularly dissolved oxygen. On raw and settled domestic sewage, for practical purposes, all of the oxygen demand is due to the first class of materials and is determined by the BOD test described below. In biologically treated effluents, a considerable proportion of the oxygen demand may be due to oxidation of class (b) compounds and will also be included in the BOD test; (c) materials present may not be included in the BOD test unless the test is based upon the calculated initial dissolved oxygen. It should be understood that all three of these classes have a direct bearing upon the oxygen balance of the waters and must be considered in the discharge of a waste to such a water. Since complete stabilization of a given waste may require a period of incubation too long for practical purposes : 5-day period has been accepted as standard. The incubation temperature has also been standardized at 20°C.

Apparatus :

Incubation bottles 250-300 ml capacity with ground glass stoppers or special BOD bottles; incubator thermostatically controlled at 20°C + 1°C.

Reagents :

Distilled water of highest purity, phosphate buffer solution, magnesium sulfate solution, calcium chloride solution, ferric chloride solution.

Procedure :

1. *Preparation of dilution water :* The distilled water used should have been stored in cotton-plugged bottles for a sufficient length of time to become saturated with DO. The water may also be aerated by shaking a partially filled bottle or with a supply of clean compressed air. The distilled water used should be as near to 20°C as possible and of the highest purity. Place the desired volume of distilled water in a suitable bottle and add 1 ml each of phosphate buffer, magnesium sulfate, calcium chloride, and ferric chloride solutions for each liter of water.

2. *Seeding :* If necessary, the dilution water is seeded by using the seed found to be the most satisfactory

for the particular waste under study. Only past experience can determine the actual amount of seed to be added per liter. Seeded dilution water should be used the same day it is made.

3. *Pretreatment :*   (a) *Samples containing caustic alkalinity or acidity :*   Neutralize to about pH 7.0 with 1 N H_2SO_4 or NaOH, using a pH meter or bromthymol blue as an outside indicator. The pH of the seeded dilution water should not be changed by the preparation of the lowest dilution of sample.

(b) *Samples containing residual chlorine compounds :*   If high concentrations of residual chlorine are present (0.1 ppm), allow to stand for 1-2 hours or until residual chlorine is dissipated. Excessive amount of residual chlorine can be neutralized by the addition of the exact concentration of sodium sulfite required.

(c) *Samples containing other toxic substances :*   Samples such as those for industrial wastes frequently require special study and treatment, for example, toxic metals derived from plating wastes.

(d) *Samples supersaturated with DO :*   Samples containing over 9 mg/l DO at 20°C may be encountered during winter months or in localities where algae are actively growing. To prevent loss of oxygen during incubation of these samples, the DO should be reduced to saturation by bringing the sample to about 20°C in a partly filled bottle and agitating it by vigorous shaking or by aerating with compressed air.

4. *Dilution technique :*   Make several dilutions of the prepared sample so as to obtain the required depletions. The following dilutions are suggested :

0.1-1.0 per cent for strong trade wastes;

1-5 per cent for raw and settled sewage;

5-25 per cent for oxidized effluents; and

25-100 per cent for polluted river waters.

Carefully siphon standard dilution water, seeded if necessary, into a graduated cylinder of 1,000 2,000 ml capacity, filling the cylinder half full without entrainment of air, Add the quantity of carefully mixed sample to make the desired dilution and dilute to the appropriate level with dilution water. Mix well with a plunger type mixing rod, avoiding entrainment of air. Siphon the mixed dilution into two BOD bottles, one for incubation and the other for determination of the initial DO in the mixture. Stopper tightly and incubate for 5-days at 20°C. The BOD bottles should be water sealed by inversion in a tray of water in the incubator or by using special water-seal bottles. Prepare succeeding dilutions of lower concentration in the same manner, or by adding dilution water to the unused portion of the preceding dilution.

5. *Determination of DO :*   If the sample represents 1 per cent or more of the lowest BOD dilution, determine DO on the undiluted sample. This determination is usually omitted on sewage and settled effluents known to have a DO content of practically zero. With samples having an immediate oxygen demand, a calculated initial DO should be used, since such a demand represents a load on the receiving water.

6. *Incubation :*   Incubate the black dilution water and the diluted samples for 5 days at 20°C. Then determine the DO in the incubated samples and the blank using the Alsterberg azide modification or the Winkler method. In special cases, other modifications may be necessary. Those dilutions showing a residual DO of at least 1 mg/l and a depletion of at least 2 mg/l should be considered the most reliable.

7. *Seed correction :*   If the dilution water is exceeded, determine the oxygen depletion of the seed by setting up a separate series of seed dilutions and selecting those resulting in 40-70 per cent oxygen depletions in 5 days. One of these depletions is then used to calculate the correction due to the small amount of seed in the dilution water. Do not use the seeded blank for seed correction because the 5-day seeded dilution water blank is subject to erratic oxidation due to the very high dilution of seed, which is not characteristic of the seeded sample.

8. *Dilution water control :* Fill two BOD bottles with unseeded, dilution water. Stopper and water-seal one of these for incubation. The other bottle is for determining the DO before incubation. The DO results on these two bottles are used as a rough check on the quality of the unseeded dilution water. The depletion obtained should not be used as a blank correction; it should not be more than 0.2 ml and preferably not more than 0.1 ml.

9. *Immediate dissolved oxygen demand :* Substances oxidizable by molecular oxygen, such as ferrous iron, sulfite, sulfide, and aldehyde, impose a load on the receiving water and must be taken into consideration. The total oxygen demand of such a substrate may be determined by using a calculated initial DO or by using the sum of the immediate dissolved oxygen demand (IDOD) and the 5 day BOD. Where a differentiation of the two components is desired, the IDOD should be determined. It should be understood that the IDOD does not necessarily represent the immediate oxidation by the iodine liberated in the acidification step of the Winkler method.

The depletion of DO in a standard water dilution of the sample in 15 min has been arbitrarily selected as the IDOD. To determine the IDOD, the DO of the sample (which in most cases is zero) and the DO of the dilution water are determined separately. An appropriate dilution of the sample and dilution water is prepared, and the DO is determined diluted samples for 5 days at 20°C. Then determine the DO in the incubated samp the DO of the dilution a load on the receiving water.

D_1 = decimal fraction of dilution water used

D_2 = decimal fraction of sample used

B_1 = DO of dilution of seed control before incubation

B_2 = DO of dilution of seed control after incubation

f = ratio of seed in sample to seed in control

$$= \frac{\% \text{ seed in } D_1}{\% \text{ seed in } B_1}$$

Seed correction = $(B_1 - B_2) \times f$

Biochemical oxygen demand

a. *When seeding is not required :*

$$\text{mg/l BOD} = \frac{D_1 - D_2}{P}$$

b. *When using seeded dilution water :*

$(D_1 - D_2) - (B_1 - B_2) \times f$

Including IDOD if small or not determined :

$$\text{mg/l BOD} = \frac{D_1 D_2}{P}$$

c. *Immediate dissolved oxygen demand :*

$$\text{mg/l IDOD} = \frac{D_0 - D_1}{P}$$

The DO determined on the unseeded dilution water after incubation is not used in the BOD calculations because this practice would overcorrect for the dilution water. In all of the above calculations, corrections are not made for small losses of DO in the dilution water during incubation. If the dilution water is unsatisfactory, proper corrections are difficult and the results are questionable.

Experiment No. 12

Object

Determination of total, suspended, dissolved and fixed solids in a sewage/water sample.

The test for solid matter is of very great importance in sewage treatment processes to indicate the physical state of the principal constituents. The ratio of the weight of suspended solids to turbidity is often referred as coefficient of fineness. The solids present in dissolved form are related to electrical conductivity.

Principle

There are two types of gravimetric analytic methods used in this experiment.

1. The substance to be determined is isolated from the other constituents in the sample by the formation of air insoluble precipitate.
2. The substance to be determined is isolated by the property of volatility.

Apparatus

Oven, crucible, muffle furnace, dessicator, weighing apparatus.

Procedure

(a) **Total solids :** Place the required quantity of the sample in a dry constant weight dish or crucible. Evaporate to dryness in an oven at 103°-105°C and dry to constant weight. Cool the dish in a dessicator. Weigh and note the increase in weight.

$$\text{Total solids (mg/L)} = \frac{(\text{weight of crucible with residue} - \text{weight of empty crucible)} \text{ mg} \times 100}{\text{ml sample}}$$

(b) **Total solids (volatile and fixed) :** Ignite the residue obtained in (a) to 600°C in a muffle furnace for 15-20 min., cool and then weigh.

$$\text{Total volatile solids (mg/L)} = \text{total solids} - \frac{(\text{weight of crucible with residue heated 600°C)} \text{ mg} \times 1000}{\text{ml sample}}$$

$$\text{Fixed solids (mg/L)} = \text{total solids} - \text{volatile solids}$$

(c) **Suspended and filtrable solids :** Filter the sample through 'Whatman' filter paper No. 44. Take a suitable quantity in a weighed dry dish/crucible. Evaporate to dryness at 103°-105°C. Cool the container to constant weight, weigh and note the increase in weight.

$$\text{Dissolved solids (mg/L)} = \frac{(\text{weight of crucible with residue} - \text{weight of empty crucible)} \text{ mg} \times 1000}{\text{ml sample}}$$

$$\text{Suspended solids} = \text{total solids (a)} - \text{filterable solids (c)}$$

Observation table

Sample details	Type of solids	Weight of		
		empty beaker	with residue	mg/L residue
	Total			
	Volatile			
	Fixed			
	Dissolved			
	Suspended			

Results

Total solids = ... mg/L
Volatile solids = ... mg/L
Fixed solids = ... mg/L
Dissolved solids = ... mg/L
Suspended solids = ... mg/L

Experiment No. 13

Object

Determination of chemical oxygen demand (COD).

Theory

The chemical oxygen demand test indicates the quantity of oxidisable materials present in water and varies with water composition, concentration of reagent, temperature, period of contact and other factors.

Chemical demand test is widely used for measuring the pollutional strength of waste waters. All organic compounds with a few exceptions can be oxidised to carbon dioxide and water by the action of strong oxidising agents regardless of biological assimilability of the substance.

Principle

Most types of organic matter are destroyed by a boiling mixture of chromic and sulphuric acids. A sample is refused with known amounts of potassium dichromate and sulhuric acid and the excess dischronate is titrated with sulphate. The amount of oxidizable organic matter, measured as oxygen equivalent, is proportional to the potassium dichromate consumed.

Apparatus

Reflux apparatus consisting of 250 ml Erlenmeyer flasks with ground glass and 300 mm jacket condensers with ground glass joint and a hot plate.

Reagents

Standard potassium dichromate 0.250 N
Sulfuric acid reagent (with 1 gm of silver sulphate in every 75 ml acid)
Ferroin indicator solution
Standard ferrous ammonium sulphate solution
Mercuric sulphate

Procedure

Standardization of titrant : Dilute 10 ml standard potassium dicaromate solution to about 100 ml. Add 30 ml conc. H_2SO_4 and allow to cool. Titrate using 2 or 3 drops (0.1-0.15 ml) ferroin indicator.

$$Normality = \frac{ml\ K_2Cr_2O_7 \times 0.25}{ml\ Fe(NH_4)_2(SO_4)_2\ used}$$

Place 0.4 g HgSO$_4$ in a refluxing flask. Add 20 ml of sample and then add 10 ml of the standard potassium dichromate solution and several pumice granules or glass beads which have been heated to 600°C for 1 hour. Slowly add 30 ml conc. H$_2$SO$_4$ containing Ag$_2$SO$_4$ through the open end of the condenser and mix thoroughly. Mix the reflux mixture thoroughly before the heat is applied.

If more chloride is present, add more HgSO$_4$ to maintain a HgSO$_4$: Cl ratio of 10 : 1.

Reflux the mixture for 2 hrs., or use a shorter period for particular wastes if it has been found to give the maximum COD. Cool and then wash the condenser with distilled water.

Dilute the mixture to about 150 ml with distilled water, cool to room temperature and titrate the excess dichromate with standard ferrous ammonium sulphate, using ferroin indicator. Generally, use 2-3 drops (0.10-0.15 ml) of indicator. Take as the end point the sharp colour change from blue green to reddish brown even though the blue green may reappear within minutes.

Reflux in the same manner a blank consisting of 20 ml distilled water together with the reagents.

Calculation

$$mg/L\ COD = \frac{(a-b)N \times 8000}{ml\ sample}$$

where
    a = ml Fe(NH$_4$)$_2$(SO$_4$)$_2$ used for blank
    b = ml Fe(NH$_4$)$_2$(SO$_4$)$_2$ used for sample
    N = normality of Fe(NH$_4$)$_2$(SO$_4$)$_2$

Observation table

Sample details	Normality of K$_2$Cr$_2$O$_7$	Amount of K$_2$Cr$_2$O$_7$ used	Normality of Fe(NH$_4$)$_2$(SO$_4$)$_2$	ml of Fe(NH$_4$)$_2$(SO$_4$)$_2$	COD mg/L

Result

COD = ... mg/L

Experiment No. 14

Object

Bacteriological examination of water.

The routine bacteriological tests are aimed at enumerating the members of the coliform group which are considered indicators of pollution. The natural habitat of these bacteria is the intestinal tract of man and other warm-blooded animals.

Another test of bacteria is aimed at detecting chemo-synthetic heterotropic heterogenous group developing under conditions of cultivation and is referred as total plate count test. This test indicates a total picture of bacteria associated with organic matter.

Apparatus and glasswares

Incubators, hot air ovens, autoclaves, colony counters, pH equipment, media preparation utensils, pipettes, graduated cylinders, pipette containers, dilution bottles or tubes, petri dishes, fermentation tubes and vials, inoculating equipment, sample bottles.

All glassware must be cleaned and sterilized (except when in metal containers).

Preparation of culture media

For the study of bacteria, it is necessary to grow them. The substances upon which the bacteria are grown are designated as culture media.

Procedure

(a) **Nutrient agar :** Add 3 gm beef extract and 5 gm peptone to a litre of distilled water. Heat slowly, preferably on a water bath, until dissolved. Adjust the pH reaction at 7.0. Then add 15 gm of agar to flask and boil. Distribute 10 ml each in test tubes and sterilise.

(b) **MacConkey's broth :** Dissolve 10 gm lactose, 20 gm peptone and 5 gm sodium chloride in 500 ml distilled water. Dissolve 5 gm bill salt in 200 ml distilled water separately. Mix the two and make up the volume to 975 ml. Adjust the pH to 7.4. Add 1.0 ml of 1% alcoholic solution of bromcresol purple. Make up the volume to 1.0 litre. Distribute in test tubes 10 ml each with fermentation tubes, plug with cotton and sterilise.

If strength of inoculum is 10 ml then dissolve the ingredients in half the volume of water (double strength).

Alternatively commercially prepared dehydrated culture media may be used.

Estimation of bacterial numbers

1. **Total count :** Place three or four sterilised nutrient agar tubes in a water bath and heat to liquefy agar. Cool to 45°C. Put 1.0, 0.1 and 0.01 ml in the molten nutrient agar and pour in sterilized petridishes. Quantities smaller than 1.0 can be secured by preparing dilution in sterilized distilled water. Let the agar solidify. Invert the petridish and incubate at 37°C for 24 hours. Count the colonies developing using a counter.

The number of colonies in a particular dish multiplied by the reciprocal of the fraction of the ml inoculated gives the number of bacteria per ml. The plates with colonies between 3 and 300 should be regarded as satisfactory.

2. **Coliform MPN (most probable number) :** Inoculate the sample in exponential order in 3 tubes each of MacConkey's broth. Use double strength tubes for 10 ml portions and single strength for 1.0 ml and 0.1 fractions. Incubate for 24 ± 2 hrs. at 35°C ± 0.5°C. Note the number of positive tubes where positivity is determined by the change in colour from purple to yellow and accumulation of gas in fermentation tube. Find out the 24 hours presumptive MPN from the MPN table. Further incubate the tubes for 24 hours and note the positive tubes. Record the 48 hour MP confirmed coliform MPN.

MPN table

Number of tubes giving positive reaction			MPN index per 100 ml
3 of 10 ml	3 of 1 ml	3 of 0.1 ml	
0	0	1	3
0	1	0	3
1	0	0	4
1	0	1	7
1	1	0	7
1	1	1	11
1	2	0	11
2	0	0	9
1	0	1	14
2	1	0	15
2	1	1	20
2	2	0	21
2	2	1	28
3	0	0	23
3	0	1	39
3	0	2	64
3	1	0	43
3	1	1	75
3	1	2	120
3	2	0	93
3	2	1	150
3	2	2	210
3	2	3	290
3	3	1	460
3	3	2	1100
3	3	3	2400

Observation table

Sample details	Counts in plate	Counts/ml

MPN	24 hrs. results				48 hrs. results			
	10 ml	1.0 ml	0.1 ml	Presumptions	10 ml	1.0 ml	0.1 ml	Confirmed

Results

Total count = ,......../ml
MPN = .../100 ml

Experiment No. 15

Object

Air pollution—Testing and instrumentation

The collection of an accurate and adequate sample from a gaseous medium presents a variety of complicated situations. Various testing procedures and instruments are employed to deal with these situations.

Sampling is done using sampling trains (EPA type) or tape samples. Particulates and gases can be sampled using tape samplers. Generally, grab sampling using vacuum pump serves the purpose for demonstrative or basic experiments.

Analysis is done using instruments which work on various principles viz. thermal conductivity, infrared rays, ultraviolet rays, colorimetry and chromatography. The instrument is chosen taking into account several factors by an expert in the field.

Analysis of inorganic particles (Ring oven method)

The ring oven method is simple, reliable and inexpensive. This method can be applied in the field as well as in the laboratory. Sampling is done with a tape sampler because of the sensitivity of the ring oven.

The detection and determination of the constituents of inorganic air pollutants is accomplished through the use of extremely sensitive organic reagents that are either specific or selective through the proper use of masking agents or through conditioning process.

General procedure

Place a piece of filter paper on the heated surface of the ring oven and introduce soluble sample material at the exact centre of the paper.

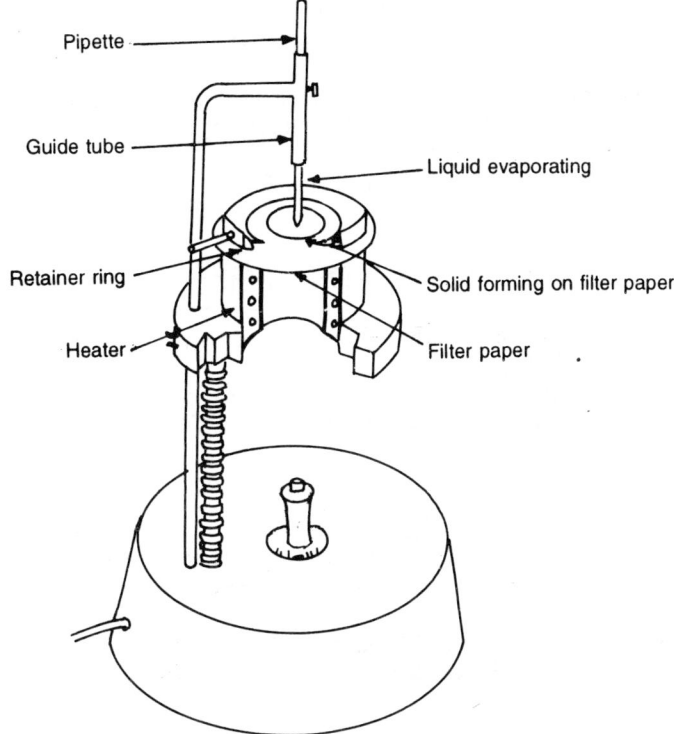

Features of ring oven.

Step 1 : Introduction
of sample

Step 2 : Transfer
and concentration

Step 3 : Analysis

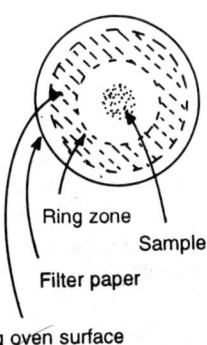

Ring zone
Sample
Filter paper

Ring oven surface
(Hot — 100°C to 110°C)

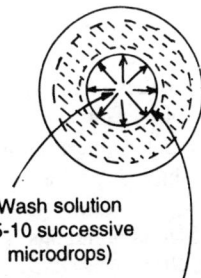

Wash solution
(5-10 successive
microdrops)

Solute (sample deposits
or solvent evaporates

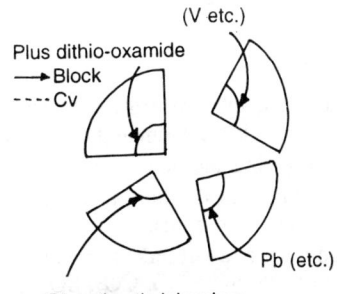

(V etc.)

Plus dithio-oxamide
→ Block
---- Cv

Pb (etc.)

Plus dimethylglyoxime
and NH_3 — red
Ni

Ring oven procedure steps.

The sample solution is washed through appropriate solvent (5-10 µl) to transport the solute to the heating surface.

As the solution approaches the heating ring zone, the carrier solvent is evaporated, thus depositing the solute as a sharply defined ring.

The filter paper with the ring of the deposited salts (sample) is finally removed from the surface of the ring oven and appropriate tests are then run on the sectors of the sample ring. The filter paper is ordinarily out into as many segments as there are tests or determinations to be run.

Testing procedures for a few pollutants are described below :

Beryllium

1. Spray ring with morin (3,5,7, 2′,4′-pentahydroxy flavone saturated in methanol) or rub with reagent crayon and heat with hot air.
2. Place the treated test paper in bath (NH₄OH-methanol, 1 : 1) for 5 minutes and dry.
3. Observe under UV radiation—yellow green fluorescence.

Sample : From sample tape, direct dissolution and transfer. Dissolved by adding 30 µl NH_4 acetate (15%), wash to ring zone with water followed by 30 µl EDTA (0.1 M).

Lead

1. Spray with dithiazone (0.005% in Cl_4).
2. Immerse paper in wash solution (0.2% KCN and 2% NH_4OH) for 1 minute.
3. Wash paper in water and press between filter papers to remove excess water. Dry in warm air—brick red ring.

Sample : Dissolution by addition of 30 µl NH_4 acetate (15%) and 30 µl $Na_2S_2O_3$ (5%) and washing to ring zone with distilled water. Another 30 µl NH_4 acetate (15%) + 30 µl KCN (0.5%) is added and washed to the ring zone with distilled water.

Analysis of inorganic particles by spectrophotometer method

This method of analysis is usually rapid and simple but the cost of the equipment is high. It is a reliable and specific method.

The procedure for determination of lead gives an idea of the method.

1. Ash samples in HNO_3, then dissolve residue in 1% HNO_3 and treat solution with hydroxylamine hydro-chloride. With careful adjustment of pH, add NH_4CN and extract with $CHCl_3$ solution of dithiazone. Repeat extraction and measure absorbance at 510 nm.

Sample : Collect particulate 1 on membrane filter (100 litres/m) or by means of electrostat precipitation. A standard containing 75 ml of 1 N HNO_3 may also be used at sampling rate of 30 litres/m.

Analysis of gaseous pollutants

Gaseous pollutants like ozone, carbon oxides, oxides of nitrogen cause health hazards. The concentration of these pollutants should be estimated to provide control measures.

Stack testing and monitoring can be done to determine emission characteristics and quantities at a particular time.

Sampling can be done using sampling train (EPA type) or tape samplers. Grab or absorption or adsorptio sampling may also be used.

Commercial analysers are available for gaseous pollutants. NDIR analysers which work with infrared rays can be used to determine CO, CO_2, SO_2, CH_4 and NH_3.

Reference for Public Health Engineering Laboratory

1. Kulkarni G.J., A Text Book of Water Supply and Sanitary Engineering, United Book Corporation, Poona, 8th edition, 1969.
2. Hussain S.K., A Text Book of Water Supply and Sanitary Engineering (in MKS), Oxford and IBH Press, New Delhi, 2nd edition, 1976.
3. Kshirsagar S.R., Water Supply Engineering, Roorkee Publishing House, Roorkee, 4th edition, 1969.
4. Mathur R.P., Water and Waste Water Testing : A Laboratory Manual, Nemchand and Bros, Roorkee, 1st edition, 1982.
5. Camp, Thomas R., Water and its Impurities, Strodsberg, Pennsylvania, Dowdan, Hutchinson and Ross, 2nd edition, 1972.
6. Lamb, James C., Water Quality and its Control, Wiley Eastern Co. Ltd., New York, 3rd edition, 1985.
7. American Water Works Association, Water Quality and Treatment : A Handbook of Public Water Supply, McGraw Hill Book Co. Ltd., New York, 2nd edition, 1966.

APPENDIX

```
0001 PROGRAM EXPONE (INPUT, OUTPUT)
0002 (*THIS PROGRAM CALCULATES TERMINAL VELOCITY FOR A GIVEN*)
0003 (*PARTICLE AND VERIFIES STOKE'S LAW*)
0004 VAR
0005 A, B, C, D, E : ARRAY [1 ..10] OF REAL
0006 DIA 1, DIA 2, DIA 3, DIA, VOL, WEIGHT, DENSITY, DISTP, TIME : REAL;
0007 GAMAF, GAMAS, MUE, SQDIA , PERDIF, AVCAL, AVCAT, VCAL, VACT : REAL
0008 I, J : INTEGER
0009 K : BOOLEAN;
0010 BEGIN
0011 I = 1
0012 K = FALSE
0013 WRITELN ('PLEASE' GIVE ALL VALUES IN SI UNITS)
0014 WRITELN
0015 WRITE ('PLEASE' ENTER OBSERVATION VALUES (<10>)
0016 READLN (J)
0017 WRITELN
0018 IF (J < = 0) OR (J) 10) THEN
0019 WRITELN ('SORRY' PROGRAM IS RESTRICTED TO TEN OBSERVATIONS ONLY)
0020 ELSE
0021 BEGIN
0022 WRITELN
0023 WRITELN ('SPECIFY THE FOLLOWING VALUES')
0024 WRITELN
0025 WRITE ('SPECIFIC WEIGHT OF LIQUID')
0026 READLN (GAMAF)
0027 WRITELN
0028 WRITE ('VISCOSITY OF LIQUID)
0029 READLN (MUE)
0030 WRITELN
0031 WHILE (I < = J) DO
0032 BEGIN
0033 WRITE ('DIA 1)
0034 READLN (DIA 1)
0035 WRITE (DIA 2)
```

```
0036 READLN (DIA 2)
0037 WRITE (DIA 3)
0038 READLN (DIA 3)
0039 WRITE ('WEIGHT OF SOLID)
0040 READLN (WEIGHT)
0041 WRITELN
0042 WRITE (DISTANCE TRAVELED BY THE SPHERE
0043 READLN (DISTP)
0044 WRITELN
0045 WRITE (TIME TAKEN)
0046 READLN (TIME)
0048 (DIA) = (DIA) + DIA
0049 ([1]) = DIA
0050 SODIA = (DIA * DIA)
0051 VOL =(22 * DIA * SODIA) / 42
0052 E [1] = VOL
0053 DENSITY = (WEIGHT / VOL)
0054 GRAMS = (9.81 * DENSITY)
0055 D [1] = GRAMS
0056 VCAL = (GRAMS - GAMAF) / (18 * MUE) * SODIA
0057 VACT = (DISTP/TIME)
0058 A [1] = VCAL
0059 B [I] = VACT
0060 I = I + 1
0061 END
0062 I = 1
0063 AVCAL = 0
0064 AVACT = 0
0065 WHILE (I < = J) DO
0066 BEGIN
0067 AVCAL = AVCAL + A [1]
0068 AVACT = AVACT + B [1]
0069 I = I + 1
0070 END
0071 AVCAL = (AVCAL/J)
0072 AVACT = (AVACT/J)
0073 PERDIF = (AVCAL - AVACT)
0074 IF (PERDIF (o) THEN
0075 PERDIF = (-PERDIF/AVACT) * 100
0076 IF (PERDIF < = 5) THEN
0077 K = TRUE
0078 WRITELN
0079 WRITE
```

```
0080 WRITELN
0081 WRITE S.No. DIA VOLUME GAMAS
0082 WRITELN VCAL VCAT REMARK
0083 WRITE
0084 WRITELN
0085 I = 1
0086 WHILE (I < = J) DO
0087 BEGIN
0088 WRITE ( 2,1 : 2)3, C [1] : 9 : 3 4, E [I] ( : 3
0089 WRITELN ( 4, D [I] 9 : 3 4, A [I] 9 : 3 4, B [I] 9 : 3
0090 WRITE
0091 WRITELN
0092 I = I + 1
0093 END
0094 IF K THEN
0095 WRITELN ('STROKE'S LAW IS VERIFIED')
0096 ELSE
0097 WRITE (INCORRECT OBSERVATIONS, EXPERIMENT IS REQUIRED TO)
0098 WRITELN (BE REPEATED WITH GREATER ACCURACY)
0099 END
0100 END


0001 PROGRAM EXPTWO (INPUT, OUTPUT)
0002 (* THIS PROGRAM CALCULATIONS THE TOTAL HEAD OF FLOW FOR A *)
0003 (* SECTION OF PIPE AND VERIFIES BERNOULLI's EQUATION *)
0004 VAR
0005 (* LIST OF VARIABLES *)
0006 PHARR, THARR, VHARR, VFARR, ARRAY, [1 5,1 6] OF REAL
0007 A, PH, VF, VH, TH, THAVG, ARRAY, [1 .. 6] OF REAL
0008 LT, WT, AT, TC, RT, DW, FR, PERDIF, REAL
0009 BOOL ARRAY [1..5] OF REAL
0010 L I J INTEGER
0011 DONE BOOL [L] : BOOLEAN
0012 BEGIN
0013 FOR L = 1 TO 6 DO
0014 BEGIN
0015 THAVG [L] = 0
0016 END
0017 FOR L = 1 TO 5 DO
0018 BOOL [L] = TRUE
```

```
0019 WRITELN (PLEASE SPECIFY THE FOLLOWING VALUES)
0020 WRITELN (PLEASE GIVE ALL VALUES IN SI UNITS)
0021 WRITE (AREA OF CONDUIT OF PEIZOMETRIC POINTS)
0022 READLN (A [1], A [2], A [3], A [4], A [5], A [6]
0023 WRITELN
0024 WRITE (LENGTH OF TANK)
0025 READLN (LT)
0026 WRITELN
0027 WRITE (PLEASE GIVE WIDTH OF TANK)
0028 READLN (WT)
0029 WRITELN
0030 AT = LT * WT
0031 I = 1
0032 WHILE (I < = 5) DO
0033 BEGIN
0034 WRITE (PLEASE GIVE TIME OF COLLECTION)
0035 READLN (TC)
0036 WRITELN
0037 WRITE (PLEASE GIVE RISE OF WATER IN TANK)
0038 READLN (rt)
0039 WRITELN
0040 WRITE (PLEASE GIVE PEIZOMETRIC HEADS AT SECTION 1,2,3,4,5,6)
0041 WRITE (PLEASE SPECIFY THE HEADS IN THE SAME SEQUENCE AS)
0042 WRITELN (THAT OF AREA OF CONDUIT AT PEIZOMETRIC SECTION)
0043 READLN (PH [1], PH [2], PH [3], PH [4], PH [5], PH [6])
0044 WRITELN
0045 DW = AT * RT
0046 FR = DW / TC
0047 J = 1
0048 A [I] = FR
0049 WHILE (J < = 6) DO
0050 BEGIN
0051 VF [J] = (FR / [J])
0052 VH [J] = (VF [J] * VF [J] / (2 * 9.81)
0053 TH [J] = VH [J] + PH [J]
0054 PHARR, J] = PH [J]
0055 VHARR [I, J] = VH [J]
0056 VFARR [I, J] = VF [J]
0057 THARR [I, J] = TH [J]
0058 J = J + 1
0059 END
0060 FOR L = 1 TO 6 DO
0061 BEGIN
```

```
0062THAVG [I] = THARR [I, L] = THAVG [I]
0063 END
0064 THAVG [I] THAVG [I] / 6
0065 PERDIT = (THAVG [I] * S / 100
0066 FOR L = 1 TO 6 DO
0067 BEGIN
0068 IF (THARR [I,L] (THAVG [I] - PERDIF) OR
0069 (THARR [I, L] (THAVG [L] + PERDIF) THEN
0070 BOOL [I] = FALSE
0071 END
0072 (* PRINT THE OUTPUT*)
0073 WRITELN
0074 WRITELN (******** TABLE OF CALCULATION *********)
0075 WRITELN
0076 WRITE
0077 WRITELN
0078 WRITE (S. NO., S, 'DISCHARGE' S, PEIZOMETRIC TABLE NO. 10)
0079 WRITE (1, 10, 2, 0, 3, 10, 4, 10, 5, 10)
0080 WRITELN ( 6, 5)
0081 WRITELN (23 CROSS SECTIONAL AREA)
0082 WRITE
0083 WRITELN
0084 FOR I = 1 TO 5 DO
0085 BEGIN
0086 WRITE (2, 1 6, A [1] 9 : 4, 5, VELOCITY 14 VF [J] : 7 : 3
0087 WRITE (4 VFARR [I,1] 7 : 3 4, VRAFF [1,2] 7 : 3 4, VFARR [ I, 3] 7 : 3)
0088 WRITELN ( 4, VFARR [I, 4] 7 : 3 , 4, VFARR [I, 5] 7 : 3, 20
0089 WRITE (23 VELOCITY HEAD 9, VHARR [I, I] 7 : 3 4, VHARR [1,2] 7 : 3
0090 WRITE (4 VHARRI [I,3] 7 : 3 4, VHARR [1,4] : 7 : 3 4, VHARR [i, 5] 7 : 3
0091 WRITELN ( 2)
0092 WRITE (23 PEIZOMETRIC HEAD 6, PHARR [I,I] 7 : 3 4)
0093 WRITE (PHARR [1, 2] 7 : 3 4, PHARR [1,3] 7 : 3 4, PHARR [1,4] 7 : 3
0094 WRITELN (4, PHARR [I,S] 7 : 3 2
0095 WRITE (23 TOTAL HEAD 12 TFARR [I, 1] 7 : 3 4, THARR [1,2] 7 : 3
0096 WRITE (4, PHARR [I, 3] 773 4, PHARR [I, 4] 773 5,, PHARR [I, 5] 7 : 3
0097 WRITELN
0098 WRITE
0099 WRITELN
0100 END
0101 L = 1
0102 DONE = TRUE
0103 WHILE (L < 6) DO
0104 BEGIN
```

```
0105 IF BOOL [L] THEN
0106 L = L + 1
0107 ELSE
0108 L = 6
0109 NED
0110 WRITELN
0111 WRITELN (******** R E S U L T ********)
0112 WRITELN
0113 WRITELN
0114 IF DONE THEN
0115 BEGIN
0116 WRITE (THE TOTAL HEAD FOR A PARTICULAR DISCHARGE IS CONSTANT)
0117 WRITELN (HENCE BERNOULLI'S THEOREM IS PROVED)
0118 END
0119 ELSE
0120 BEGIN
0121 WRITELN
0122 WRITE (INCORRECT OBSERVATIONS, EXPERIMENT IS REQUIRED TO BE)
0123 WRITELN (REPEATED WITH GREATER ACCURACY)
0124 END
0125 END
```

```
0001 PROGRAM EXPTHREE (INPUT, OUTPUT)
0002 (* THIS PROGRAM CALCULATES DARCY'S FRICTION FACTOR OF)
0003 (* PIPES OF DIFFERENT DIAMETER*)
0004 (*THIS PROGRAM IS WRITTEN FOR 5 DIFFERENT DIAMETERS AND *)
0005 (* EACH DIAMETER HAVING 3 DIFFERENT DISCHARGES*)
0006 VAR
0007 (* LIST OF VARIABLES*)
0008 D, L : ARRAY [1 ..5] OF REAL
0009 T, H 1, H 2, H 3, VOL, Q, VF, F, ARRAY [1 ..5, 1..3] OF REAL
0010 ROHG, ROW, FTOTAL, AVGF, REAL
0011 I, J, K, INTEGER
0012 BEGIN
0013 WRITELN (PLEASE GIVE THE FOLLOWING VALUES)
0014 WRITELN
0015 WRITELN (PLEASE SPECIFY ALL THE VALUES IS SI UNITS)
0016 WRITELN
0017 (*READ THE INPUT*)
0018 WRITE (MASS DENSITY OF MANOMETER FLUID)
```

```
0019 READLN (ROHG)
0020 WRITELN
0021 WRITE (MASS DENSITY OF WATER)
0023 WRITELN
0024 I = 1
0025 WRITE (PLEASE GIVE THE NO. OF DIFFERENT DIAMETER PIPES)
0026 READLN (K)
0027 WRITELN
0028 IF (K < = 0) OR (k . 5) THEN
0029 WRITE (SORRY PROGRAM IS RESTRICTED TO 5 DIFFERENT)
0030 WRITELN (DIAMETER OBSERVATIONS ONLy)
0031 FISE
0032 BEGIN
0033 WHILE (i < = k) DO
0034 BEGIN
0035 WRITE (PLEASE GIVE DIA OF PIPES)
0036 READLN (d [I])
0037 WRITELN
0038 WRITE (PLEASE GIVE LENGTH OF PIPES BETWEEN PRESSURE TAPPINGS
0039 READLN (l [I])
0040 WRITELN
0041 I = I + 1
0042 END
0043 FOR I - 1 TO K DO
0044 FOR J = 1 TO 3 DO
0045 FTOTAL = 0
0046 BEGIN
0047 WRITE (PLEASE GIVE TIME OF COLLECTION)
0048 FOR I = 1 TO K DO
0049 FOR J = 1 TO 3 DO
0050 BEGIN
0051 READLN (t [I,J]
0052 WRITELN
0053 END
0054 WRITE (PLEASE GIVE MANOMETER READINGS)
0055 FOR I = 1 TO K DO
0056 FOR J = 1 TO 3 DO
0057 BEGIN
0058 READLN (H 3 [I, J]
0059 WRITELN
0060 END
0061 WRITE (PLEASE GIVE MANOMETER READINGS, H 1 )
0062 FOR I = 1 TO K DO
```

```
0063 FOR J = 1 TO 3 DO
0064 BEGIN
0065 READLN (h 1 [I, J]
0066 WRITELN
0067 END
0068 WRITE (PLEASE GIVE DISCHARGE COLLECTED)
0069 FOR I = 1 TO K DO
0070 FOR J = 1 TO 3 DO
0071 BEGIN
0072 READLN (VOL [ I, J]
0073 WRITELN
0074 END
0075 (*START CALCULATION*)
0076 H 2 [I,J] = (H 3 [I,J] - H 1 [I, J])
0077 HF [I,J] = (ROHG - ROW) / ROW) * H 2 [I, J]
0078 Q [I,J] = (VOL [I, J) / T [I, J]
0079 VF [I,J] = (22 * Q [I,J] / (28 * D [I]) / (L [I] * VF [I,J] * VF [I,J]
0080 F [I,J] = (2 * 9.81 * HF [I,J] D [I]) / (L [I] * VF [I,J] * VF [I, J]
0081 FTOTAL = FTOTAL + F [I,J]
0082 END
0083 AVGF = FTOTAL / (3 * K)
0084 (* START PRINTING*)
0085 WRITELN
0086 WRITELN TABLE OF RESULTS
0087 WRITELN
0088 WRITELN
0089 WRITE
0090 WRITELN
0091 WRITE ( S. NO. 10, DIA, 20, VALUES 20 1, 10)
0092 WRITELN (2 10 3 10
0093 WRITE
0094 WRITELN
0095 I = 1
0096 WHILE (I < = k) DO
0097 BEGIN
0098 WRITE (2, i 1,
0099 WRITELN
0100 WRITE
0101 WRITELN
0102 WRITE
0103 WRITELN
0104 WRITE
0105 WRITELN
```

```
0106 WRITE
0107 WRITELN
0108 I = I + 1
0109 END
0110 WRITELN
0111 WRITELN
0112 WRITELN (DARCY'S FRICTION FACTOR "F" = AVGF : 9 : 3)
0113 END
```

```
0001 PROGRAM EXPFOUR (INPUT, OUTPUT)
0002 (*tHIS PROGRAM CALCULATES THE COEFFICIENT OF DISCHARGE*)
0003 (*VELOCITY CONTRACTION AND RESISTANCE FOR AN OFFICE*)
0004 (*UNDER CONSTANT HEAD AND WRITES THEM IN TABULAR FORM*)
0005 CONST
0006 PI = 3.1456
0007 G = 9.81
0008 (*LIST OF VARIABLES*)
0009 VAR
0010 A, B, C, D, E, F, G, H, M : ARRAY [1...10] OF REAL
0011 X, Y, V, ARRAY [1 ...3] OF REAL
0012 DO, LT, WT, AT, AO, DW, RW, TC, VC, HW, VTH, REAL
0013 CV, VOL, Q, QTH, CD, CC, AVCV, AVCC, AVCR, REAL
0014 I, J, K : INTEGER
0015 BEGIN
0016 i = 1
0017 (*READ THE INPUT*)
0018 WRITELN ('PLEASE PROVIDE ALL THE VALUES IN SI UNITS')
0019 WRITELN
0020 WRITE ('PLEASE FURNISH THE OBSERVATION VALUES')
0021 READLN (J)
0022 IF (J < = 0 OR (J) 10) THEN
0023 BEGIN
0024 WRITELN ('SORRY' PROGRAM IS RESTRICTED TO TEN OBSERVATIONS ONLY')
0025 END
0026 ELSE
0027 BEGIN
0028 WRITELN
0029 WRITELN (SPECIFY THE FOLLOWING VALUES)
0030 WRITELN
0031 WRITE (DIA OF ORIFICE)
```

```
0032 READLN (DO)
0033 WRITELN
0034 WRITE (LENGTH OF MEASURING TANK)
0035 READLN (LT)
0036 WRITELN
0037 WRITE (WIDTH OF MEASURING TANK)
0038 READLN (WT)
0039 WRITELN
0040 AT = LT * WT
0041 AO = (PI * SQR DO)/ 4
0042 WHILE (I < = J) DO
0043 BEGIN
0044 WRITE (X CO-ORDINATE OF THE JET)
0045 FOR K = 1 TO 3 DO
0046 BEGIN
0047 READLN (X [K])
0048 WRITELN
0049 END
0050 WRITE (Y CO-ORDINATE OF THE JET)0051 FOR K = 1 TO 3 DO
0051 FOR K = 1 TO 3 DO
0052 BEGIN
0053 READLN (Y [K])
0054 WRITELN
0055 END
0056 WRITE (INITIAL DEPTH OF WATER IN MEASURING TANK)
0057 READLN (DW)
0058 WRITELN
0059 WRITE (FINAL DEPTH OF WATER IN MEASURING TANK)
0060 READLN (RW)
0061 WRITELN
0062 WRITE (TIME OF COLLECTION)
0063 READLN (TC)
0064 WRITELN
0065 FOR K = 1 TO 3 DO
0066 V = 0
0067 BEGIN
0068 V [K] = SQRT (G * SQR X [K] / (4 * Y [K])
0069 V = V + V[K]
0070 END
0071 VC = V/3
0072 A [I] = VC
0073 HW = RW   DW
0074 B [I] = HW
```

```
0075 VTH = SQRT (2 * G * HW)
0076 C [I] = VTH
0077 CV = V/VTH
0078 D[I] = CV
0079 VOL = AT * HW
0080 Q = VOL/TC
0081 E [I] = Q
0082 QTH = AO * VTH
0083 F [I] = QTH
0084 CD = Q/QTH
0085 G [I] = CD
0086 CC = CD/CV
0087 H [I] = CC
0088 CR = (1/ (SQR CV) - 1)
0089 M [I] = CR
0090 I = I + 1
0091 END
0092 I = 1
0093 AVCV = 0
0094 AVCD = 0
0095 AVCC = 0
0096 AVCR = 0
0097 WHILE (I < = J) DO
0098 BEGIN
0099 AVCV = AVCV + D [I]
0100 AVCD = AVCD + G [I]
0101 AVCC = AVCC + H [I]
0102 AVCR = AVCR + M [I]
0103 I = I + 1
0104 END
0105 AVCV = (AVCV/J)
0106 AVCD = (AVCD/J)
0107 AVCC = (AVCC/J)
0108 AVCR = (AVCR/J)
0109 (*START PRINTING*)
0110 WRITELN (********* TABLE OF CALCULATION *********)
0111 WRITELN
0112 WRITELN
0113 WRITELN
0114 WRITE
0115 WRITELN
0116 WRITE (S.NO. V H VTH CV Q)
0117 WRITELN (OTH CD CC CR)
```

```
0118 WRITE
0119 WRITELN
0120 I = 1
0121 WHILE (I < = J) DO
0122 BEGIN
0123 WRITE (2, I : 2, 2, A [I] : 6 : 3, 3, B [I] : 6 : 3, 3, C [I] : 6 : 3
0124 WRITE (3, D [I] 6 : 6, 4, E [I] 6 : 3, 3, F [I] : 6 : 3, 3, G [I] : 6 : 3)
0125 WRITE (6 : 3, 4, H [I] : 6 : 3, 4, M [I] : 6 : 3)
0126 WRITE
0127 WRITELN
0128 I = I + 1
0129 END
0130 WRITELN
0131 WRITELN
0132 WRITELN (***********)
0133 WRITELN ( * R E S U L T * )
0134 WRITELN
0135 WRITELN
0136 WRITELN
0137 WRITELN
0138 WRITELN (AVERAGE VALUE OF COEFFICIENT OF VELOCITY = AVCV : 10 : 4)
0139 WRITELN
0140 WRITELN (AVERAGE VALUE OF COEFFICIENT OF DISCHARGE = AVCD : 10 : 4)
0141 WRITELN
0142 WRITELN (AVERAGE VALUE OF COEFFICIENT OF CONTRACTION = AVCC : 10 : 4)
0143 WRITELN
0144 WRITELN (AVERAGE VALUE OF COEFFICIENT OF RESISTANCE = AVCR : 10 : 4)
0145 END
0146 END
```

```
0001 PROGRAM EXPFIVE (INPUT, OUTPUT)
0002 (*THIS PROGRAM CALCULATES THE COEFFICIENT OF DISCHARGE*)
0003 (*VELOCITY CONTRACTION AND RESISTANCE FOR AN OFFICE*)
0004 (*UNDER CONSTANT HEAD AND WRITES THEM IN TABULAR FORM*)
0005 CONST
0006 P I = 3. 1456
0007 G = 9.81
0008 (*LIST OF VARIABLES*)
0009 VAR
0010 A, B, C, D, E, F, G, H, M, ARRAY [1..10] OF REAL
```

```
0011 X, Y, V, ARRAY [1...3] OF REAL
0012 DO, LT, Q, QTH, CD, CC, AVCV, AVCD, AVCC, AVCR, REAL
0013 CV, VOL, Q, QTH, CD, CC, AVCV, AVCC, AVCR, REAL
0014 I, J, K INTEGER
0015 BEGIN
0016 I = 1
0017 (*READ THE INPUT*)
0018 WRITELN (PLEASE PROVIDE ALL THE VALUES IN SI UNITS)
0019 WRITELN
0020 WRITE (PLEASE FURNISH THE OBSERVATION VALUES)
0021 READLN (J)
0022 IF (J < = 0) OR (J > 10) THEN
0023 BEGIN
0024 WRITELN (SORRY, PROGRAM IS RESTRICTED TO TEN OBSERVATIONS ONLY)
0025 END
0026 ELSE
0027 BEGIN
0028 WRITELN
0029 WRITELN (SPECIFY THE FOLLOWING VALUES)
0030 WRITELN
0031 WRITE (DIA OF ORIFICE)
0032 READLN (DO)
0033 WRITELN
0034 WRITE (LENGTH OF MEASURING TANK)
0035 READLN (LT)
0036 WRITELN
0037 WRITE (WIDTH OF MEASURING TANK)
0038 READLN (WT)
0039 WRITELN
0040 AT = LT * WT
0041 AO = (PI * SQR DO)/4
0042 WHILE (I < J) DO
0043 BEGIN
0044 WRITE (X CO-ORDINATE OF THE JET)
0045 FOR K = 1 TO 3 DO
0046 BEGIN
0047 READLN (X [K])
0048 WRITELN
0049 END
0050 WRITE (Y CO-ORDINATE OF THE JET)
0051 FOR K = 1 TO 3 DO
0052 BEGIN
0053 READLN (Y [K] )
```

```
0054 WRITELN
0055 END
0056 WRITE (INITIAL DEPTH OF WATER IN MEASURING TANK)
0057 READLN (DW)
0058 WRITELN
0059 WRITE (FINAL DEPTH OF WATER IN MEASURING TANK)
0060 READLN (RW)
0061 WRITELN
0062 WRITE (TIME OF COLLECTION)
0063 READLN (TC)
0065 FOR K = 1 TO 3 DO
0066 V = 0
0067 BEGIN
0068 V [K] = SQRT (G * SQR X [K]) / (4 * Y [K])
0069 V = V + V [K]
0070 END
0071 VC = V/3
0072 A [I] = VC
0073 HW = RW - DW
0074 B [I] = HW
0075 VTH = SQRT (2 * G * HW)
0076 C [I] = VTH
0077 CV = V/VTH
0078 D [I] = CV
0079 VOL = AT * HW
0080 Q = VOL/TC
0081 E [I] = Q
0082 QTH = AO * VTH
0083 F [I] = QTH
0084 CD = Q/QTH
0085 G [I] = CD
0086 CC = CD/CV
0087 H [I] = CC
0088 CR = (1/(SQR CV) - 1)
0089 M [I] = CR
0090 I = I + 1
0091 END
0092 I = 1
0093 AVCV = 0
0094 AVCD = 0
0095 AVCC = 0
0096 AVCR = 0
0097 WHILE (I < J) DO
```

```
0098 BEGIN
0099 AVCV = AVCV + D[I]
0100 AVCD = AVCD + H[I]
0101 AVCC = AVCC + H[I]
0102 AVCR = AVCR + M[I]
0103 I = I + 1
0104 END
0105 AVCV = (AVCV/J)
0106 AVCD = (AVCD/J)
0107 AVCC = (AVCC/J)
0108 AVCR = (AVCR/J)
0109 (*START PRINTING *)
0110 WRITELN (********** TABLE OF CALCULATION *********)
0111 WRITELN
0112 WRITELN
0113 WRITELN
0114 WRITE
0115 WRITELN
0116 WRITE (S. NO. V H VTH CV Q)
0117 WRITELN (QTH CD CC CR)
0118 WRITE
0119 WRITELN
0120 I = 1
0121 WHILE (I < = J) DO
0122 BEGIN
0123 WRITE (2, I : 2, 2, A [I] : 6 : 3, 3, B [I] : 6 : 3, 3, c [I] : 6 : 3)
0124 WRITE (3, D [I] 6 : 6, 4, E[I] : 6 : 3, 3, F [I], 6 : 3, 3 : G [I] )
0125 WRITE ( 6 : 3, 4, H [I] : 6 : 3, 3, F [I] : 6 : 3, 3, G [I])
0126 WRITE
0127 WRITELN
0128 I = I + 1
0129 END
0130 WRITELN
0131 WRITELN
0132 WRITELN (*********)
0133 WRITELN (* R E S U L T *)
0134 WRITELN (******)
0135 WRITELN
0136 WRITELN
0137 WRITELN
0138 WRITELN (AVERAGE VALUE OF COEFFICIENT OF VELOCITY = AVCV : 10 : 4)
0139 WRITELN
0140 WRITELN (AVERAGE VALUE OF COEFFICIENT OF DISCHARGE = AVCD : 10 : 4)
```

0141 WRITELN
0142 WRITELN (AVERAGE VALUE OF COEFFICIENT OF CONTRACTION = AVCC : 10 : 4)
0143 WRITELN
0144 WRITELN (AVERAGE VALUE OF COEFFICIENT OF RESISTANCE = AVCR : 10 : 4)
0145 END
0146 END

0001 PROGRAM EXPSIX (INPUT, OUTPUT)
0002 (* THIS PROGRAM CALCULATES COEFFICIENT OF VELOCITY AND MOMENTUM *)
0003 (* DISTRIBUTION FOR A STEADY TURBULENT OPEN CHANNEL FLOW *)
0004 (* LIST OF VARIABLES *)
0005 VAR
0006 N, N1, Vm, Vcsqr, Vccube : ARRAY [1..3,1..5] OF REAL;
0007 T, Numb, I, J : INTEGER
0008 Hao, Hbo, Hco, Ha1, Hb1, W, H, A, delA, HW, Q : REAL
0009 Vmtotal, AVVm, AVV, Hb1, W, H, A, delA, Hw, q : REAL
0010 Veldiscoeff, Momdiscoeff, Vccubetotal, Vctotal : REAL
0011 CUAVV, SQAVV, REAL
0012 BEGIN
0013 (* READ THE INPUT *)
0014 WRITELN (PLEASE SPECIFY ALL THE VALUES IN SI UNITS)
0015 WRITELN
0016 WRITELN (PLEASE GIVE THE FOLLOWING VALUES)
0017 WRITELN
0018 WRITE (INITIAL HEAD AT A)
0019 READLN (Hao)
0020 WRITELN
0021 WRITE (INITIAL HEAD AT B)
0022 READLN (Hbo)
0023 WRITELN
0024 WRITE (INITIAL HEAD AT C)
0025 READLN (Hco)
0026 WRITELN
0027 WRITE (FINAL HEAT AT A)
0028 READLN (Ha1)
0029 WRITELN
0030 WRITE (FINAL HEAT AT B)
0031 READLN (Hb1)
0032 WRITELN
0033 WRITE (FINAL HEAT AT C)

```
0034 READLN (hC1)
0035 WRITELN
0036 WRITE (LENGTH OF THE FLOW SECTION, W)
0037 READLN (W)
0038 WRITELN
0039 WRITE (TIME, T)
0040 READLN (T)
0041 WRITELN
0042 WRITE (GIVE THE PROPELLER NOS, i.e. 1 OR 2 OR 3)
0043 READLN (nUMB)
0044 WRITE (GIVE SECTION POINT VALUES, ROW WISE, LIKE N 11, N 12, Etc.)
0045 FOR I = 1 TO 3 DO
0046 FOR J = 1 TO 5 DO
0047 BEGIN
0048 READLN (N [I,J])
0049 N1, [I,J] = [N [I,J] / T)
0050 A = H * W
0051 DELa = (A / 15)
0052 Hw = (Hco - Hc1)
0053 Q = (Hco / Hw)
0054 FOR I = 1 TO 3 DO
0055 FOR J = 1 TO 5 DO
0056 BEGIN
0057 CASE Numb OF
0058 1 : IF N1 [I, J] < = 5.33 THEN
0059 Vm [I,J] = (0.0565 * N1 [I,J] + 0.035
0060 ELSE
0061 Vm [I,J] = (0.0550 * N1 [I,J] + 0.043)
0062 2 : IF N1 [I,J] < = 1.08 THEN
0063 Vm [I,J] = (0.0943 * n1 [I,J] + 0.030
0064 ELSE
0065 Vm [I,J] = (0.1026 * N1 [I,J]) + 0.VE1)
0066 3 : IF N1 [I,Jj < 0.56 THEN
0067 Vm [I,J] = (0.2197 * N1 [I,J] + 0.030
0068 ELSE
0069 IF N1 [I,Jj 2.50 THEN
0070 Vm [I,J] = (0.2530 * N1 [I,J] + 0.005
0071 ELSE
0072 Vm [I,J] = (0.2498 * N1 [I,J] + 0.013)
0073 END (* Case of *)
0074 END
0075 Vmtotal = 0
0076 FOR I = 1 TO 3 DO
```

```
0077 FOR J = 1 TO 5 DO
0078 BEGIN
0079 Vmtotal = Vmtotal + Vm [I,J]
0080 AVVM = Vmtotal/15
0081 avv = (Q / A)
0082 SQAVV = AVV * AVV
0083 CUAVV = (SQAVV * ACC)
0084 E = (ABS (AVV - AVVm / AVV) * 100)
0085 CV = (AVV/AVVM)
0086 Vcsqrtotal = 0
0087 Vccubetotal = 0
0088 Vctotal = 0
0089 END, (*OF LOOP*)
0090 FOR I = 1 TO 3 DO
0091 FOR J = 1 TO 5 DO
0092 BEGIN
0093 Vc [I,J] = (Cv * vM [I,J]
0094 Vctotal = Vctotal + Vc [I,J]
0095 Vcsqr [I,J] = Vc [ I,J] * Vc [I,J]
0096 Vcsqrtotal = Vcsqrtotal + Vcsqr[I,J]
0097 Vccube [I,J] = (Vcsqr [I,J] * Vc [I,J]
0098 vccubetotal = Vccubetotal + Vccube [I,J]
0099 END (*OF LOOP *)
0100 END, (*OF LOOP*)
0101 (*START CALCULATION*)
0102 VELDISCOEFF = (VCCUBETOTAL / (CUAVV) * 15)
0103 MOMDISCOEFF = (VCSQRTOTAL / (SQAVV) *15)
0104 WRITELN
0105 WRITELN
0106 WRITELN (****** TABLE OF CALCULATIONS ******)
0107 WRITELN
0108 WRITELN
0109 WRITELN (TABLE FOR DIFFERENT SECTION VALUES VIZ, N11, N12, N13 etc.)
0110 WRITELN
0111 WRITE
0112 WRITELN
0113 WRITE
0114 WRITELN
0115 WRITE
0116 WRITELN
0117 FOR I = 1 TO 3 DO
0118 BEGIN
0119 WRITE
```

```
0120 WRITELN
0121 WRITE
0123 END
0124 WRITELN
0125 WRITELN
0126 WRITELN (TABLE FOR N1 = N/T)
0127 WRITELN
0128 WRITE
0130 FOR i = 1 TO 3 DO
0131 BEGIN
0132 WRITE
0133 WRITELN
0134 WRITE
0135 WRITELN
0136 END
0137 WRITELN
0138 WRITELN
0139 WRITELN (TABLE FOR V MEASURED)
0140 WRITELN
0141 WRITE
0142 WRITELN
0143 FPR I = 1 TO 3 DO
0144 BEGIN
0145 WRITE
0146 WRITELN
0147 WRITE
0148 WRITELN
0149 WRITELN
0150 WRITELN (SUM OF V MEASURED = Vmtotal : 6 : 2)
0151 WRITELN
0152 WRITELN
0153 WRITELN (TABLE FOR V CORRECTED Vc)
0154 WRITELN
0155 WRITE
0156 WRITELN
0157 FOR I = 1 TO 3 DO
0158 BEGIN
0159 WRITE
0160 WRITELN
0161 WRITE
0162 WRITELN
0163 END
0164 WRITELN
```

```
0165 WRITELN (SUM OF V CORRECTED = Vctotal : 6 : 2)
0166 WRITELN
0167 WRITELN
0168 WRITELN (TABLE FOR SQUARE OF V CORRECTED, Vc)
0169 WRITELN
0170 WRITE
0171 WRITELN
0172 FOR I = 1 TO 3 DO
0173 BEGIN
0174 WRITE (4, Vcsqr [I,J] : 6 : 2, 9, Vcsqr [I, 2] : 6 : 2, 7)
0175 WRITELN (Vcsqr [I,3] : 6 : 2, 6, Vcsqr [I,4] : 6 : 2, 8, Vcsqr [I,5]: 6 : 2)
0176 WRITE
0177 WRITELN
0178 END
0179 WRITELN
0180 WRITELN
0181 WRITELN (SUM OF SQUARE OF V CORRECTED = Vcsqrtotal : 8 : 2)
0182 WRITELN
0183 WRITELN
0184 WRITELN (TABLE FOR CUBE OF V CORRECTED, Vccube)
0185 WRITELN
0186 WRITE
0187 WRITELN
0188 FOR I = 1 TO 3 DO
0189 BEGIN
0190 WRITE (2, Vccube [I,1] : 8 : 2, 7, Vccube [1,2] : 8 : 2, 5, Vccube [1,3]
0191 WRITELN (8 : 2, 4, Vccube [1,4] : 8 : 2, 6, Vccube [1,5] : 8 : 2
0192 WRITE
0193 WRITELN
0194 END
0195 WRITELN
0196 WRITELN (SUM OF CURES OF V CORRECTED = Vccubetotal : 9 : 2)
0197 WRITELN
0198 WRITELN
0199 WRITELN (****** R E S U L T ******)
0200 WRITELN
0201 WRITELN
0202 WRITELN
0203 WRITELN (MEASURED AVERAGE VELOCITY = Avvm : 12 : 6)
0204 WRITELN
0205 WRITELN
0206 WRITELN (MEASURING ERROR = E : 6 : 3)
0207 WRITELN
```

```
0208 WRITELN
0209 WRITELN (VELOCITY CORRECTION FACTOR = CV : 12 : 6)
0210 WRITELN
0211 WRITELN
0212 WRITELN (VELOCITY DISTRIBUTION COEFFICIENT = VELDISCOEFF : 12 : 6)
0213 WRITELN
0214 WRITELN
0215 WRITELN (MOMENTUM DISTRIBUTION COEFFICIENT = MOMDISCOEFF : 12 : 6)
0216 END
```

```
0001 = PROGRAM EXPSEVEN (INPUT, OUTPUT)
0002 (*THIS PROGRAM CALCULATES ENERGY LOSS (HEAD LOSS) IN PIPES*)
0003 (*DUE TO FRICTION IN PIPE WALL, GRADUAL EXPANSION OR CONTRACTION *)
0004 (*OR CONTRACTION, SUDDEN EXPANSION OR CONTRACTION OF PIPE DIA, BENDS*)
0005 (*OBSTRUCTION ECT AND WRITES THEM DOWN IN A TABULAR FORM AND GIVES*)
0006 (*TOTAL HEAD LOSS DUE TO THE ABOVE FACTORS8)
0007 (*LIST OF VARIABLES8)
0008 CONST
0009 PI = 3.1415927, GAMMAM, 13.6 GAMMAW = 1.00
0010 TYPE
0011 POINTS = 1.37
0012 HUM = SET OF POINTS
0013 VAR
0014 NUM0, NUM1, NUM2, NUM3, NUM4, HUM
0015 I = POINTS
0016 HA, HB, DELTA, Q, D1, D2, A1, A2, V1, V2, M1, M2, A3, REAL
0017 K1, K2, K3, K4, DELHM, SUM, REAL
0018 KS, L : ARRAY [1..6] OF REAL
0019 DELH, H2, H1, Z, TVAR, H, D, F, K, HL, ARRAY [1...40] OF REAL
0020 DONE : BOOLEAN
0021 IK : INTEGER
0022 (*READ THE INPUT*)
0023 BEGIN
0024 WRITELN (PLEASE SPECIFY THE FOLLOWING VALUES)
0025 WRITELN (PLEASE FURNISH ALL THE VALUES IN CGS VALUES)
0026 NUM0 = [1,4,5,8,9,11,12,14,17,18,19,20,23,24,29,30,35]
0027 NUM1 = [1,7,8,9,13,14,16,17,18,19,20,21,22,23,24,26,28,29,30,32,34)
0028 NUM2 = [3,4,5,10,11,12]
0029 NUM3 = [2,6]
0030 NUM4 = [1,8,9,14,17,18,19,20,23,24,29,30,35)
```

```
0031 WRITELN
0032 WRITE (PLEASE ENTER HEAD AT A)
0033 READLN(HA)
0034 WRITE (PLEASE ENTER HEAD AT B)
0035 READLN(HB)
0036 DELTA = HA - HB
0037 Q = 4585 * (SQRT (DELTA)
0038 WRITELN
0039 WRITE (PLEASE ENTER DIAMETER (SMALLER)
0040 READLN (D1)
0041 WRITELN
0042 WRITE (PLEASE ENTER DIAMETER (BIGGER)
0043 READLN (D2)
0044 WRITELN
0045 (* CALCULATE AREA, VELOCITY, K1, K2, K3, K4, ETC *)
0046 A1, (PI * EXP (2 * LN (D1) / 4
0047 A2 = (PI * EXP (2 * LN (D2) / 4
0048 V1 = Q / A 1
0049 V2 = Q / A 2
0050 M 1 = (EXP (2 * LN (V1) / ( 2 * 981)
0051 M 2 = (EXP (2 * LN (V2) / (2 * 981)
0052 K 1 = D 1 / M 1
0053 K 2 = D 2 / M 2
0054 A 3 = 4 * (EXP ( 4 * LN (D1)
0055 K 3 = (A 3/ (D 2 * D2) + (D 1 * D 1) * ( D 2 + D 1) * M 2)
0056 K 4 = 1 / (EXP (2 * LN (EXP ( 2 * LN ( D 2/D 1) -1)
0057 (*CALCULATE KS*)
0058 FOR i = 1 TO 6 DO
0059 BEGIN
0060 WRITELN
0061 WRITE (PLEASE ENTER L = I : 1)
0062 READLN (L (i)
0063 KS [I] = L [I] / M1
0064 END (*OF FOR*)
0065 FOR I = 1 TO 35 DO
0066 BEGIN
0067 IF (I IN NUMO) THEN
0068 BEGIN
0069 WRITELN
0070 WRITE (PLEASE ENTER HEIGHT (Z)
0071 READLN (Z [I])
0072 WRITELN
0073 WRITE (PLEASE ENTER h1)
```

```
0074 READLN (H 1 [I])
0075 WRITELN
0076 WRITE (PLEASE ENTER h2)
0077 READLN (H2 [I])
0078 DELH [I] = H2 [I] - H1 [I]
0079 TVAR [I] = DELH [I] * (GAMMAM / GAMMAW)
0080 ELSE
0081 IF (I IN NUMA) THEN
0082 H [I] = M 1 + (H1 [I] + TVAR [I])
0083 ELSE
0084 H[I] = M2 + (H1 [I] + TVAR [I])
0085 END (*OF IF*)
0086 IK = 0
0087 DONE = FALSE
0088 WHILE (NOT DONE) DO
0089 BEGIN
0090 IK = IK + 1
0091 IF (1 - IK) IN NUMO0 THEN
0092 DONE = TRUE
0093 END, (*OF WHILE*)
0094 IF (IK = 1)THEN
0095 HL [I - IK] = H [I] - H [IK]
0096 ELSE
0097 DELHH = H [I] - H [IK]
0098 END (*OF FOR*)
0099 FOR I = 1 TO 34 DO
0100 BEGIN
0101 WRITELN
0102 WRITE (PLEASE ENTER DISTANCE BETWEEN 1 : 3, AND (1 + 1) : 3
0103 READLN (D [I])
0104 END; (*OF FOR*)
0105 (*CALCULATE HEAD DIFFERENCE BETWEEN TWO SECTIONS*)
0106 HL [I] = HL [8] * D [I]/D[8]
0107 HL [3] = HL [4] * D [3]/D[4]
0108 HL [2] = H[4] - H[1] - HL[1] - HL[4]
0109 HL [5] = HL [4] * D [5] / D [4]
0110 HL [7] = HL [8] * D [7] / D [8]
0111 HL [6] = H [8] - H [5] - HL [7] - HL [5]
0112 HL [10] = HL [1] * D [10] / D [11]
0113 HL [12] = HL [11] * D [12] / D [11]
0114 HL [9] = H [1] - H [10] - HL [10]
0115 HL [13] = H [14] - H [12] - HL [12]
0116 HL [20] = HL [19] * D [20] / D [19]
```

```
0117 HL [22] = HL [23] D [22] / D [23]
0118 HL [21] = H [23] - H [20] - HL [20] - HL 22
0119 HL [24] = H [23] * D [24] / D [23]
0120 HL [28] = HL [29] * D [28] / D [29]
0121 HL [25] = H [28] - H [24] - HL [24] - HL [28]
0122 HL [14] = HL [13] * D [12] / D [13]
0123 HL [16] = HL [17] * D [16] / D [17]
0124 HL [15] = H [17] - H [14] - HL [14] - HL [16]
0125 HL [34] = HL [29] * D [34] / D [ 29]
0126 HL [32] = HL [34] * D [32] / D [34]
0127 HL [26] = HL [29] * D [26] / D [29]
0128 HL [30] = HL [29] * D [26] / D [29]
0129 HL [31] = (1/2) * (H [35] - H [30] - HL [03] - HL [32] - HL [34])
0130 HL [32] HL [29] * D 32] / D [29]
0131 HL [34] = HL [31]
0132 HL [34] = HL [29] * D [34] / D [29]
0133 HL [35] = H [9] - H [11] - HL [9] - HL [10]
0134 HL [36] = H [12] - H [14] - HL [12] - HL [13]
0135 FOR I = 1 TO 36 DO
0136 BEGIN
0137 SUM = 0
0138 IF (1 IN NUMI) THEN
0139 K [I] = K 1
0140 ELSE
0141 IF (I IN NUM2) THEN
0142 K [I] = K 2
0143 ELSE
0144 IF (I IN NUM3) THEN
0145 K [I] = K 3
0146 ELSE
0147 BEGIN
0148 CASE I OF
0149 15 : K[I] = KS [1]
0150 21 : K[I] = KS [2]
0151 25 : K[I] = KS [3]
0152 27 : K[I] = KS [4]
0153 31 : K[I] = KS [5]
0154 33 : K[I] = KS [6]
0155 END
0156 F[I] = HL[I] * K[I] / D[I]
0157 SUM = SUM + F[I]
0158 END
0159 K[35] = K4
```

```
0160 K[37] = K4
0161 F[36] = HL[I] * K[I]
0162 F[37] = HL[I] * K[I]
0163 SUM = SUM + F[36] + F [37]
0164 WRITELN
0165 WRITELN (A) CALCULATION OF DISCHARGE AND VELOCITIES
0166 WRITELN
0167 WRITELN (DISCHARGE)
0168 WRITELN
0169 WRITELN (HA = HB 0 : 2)
0170 WRITELN (HB = HB 0 : 2)
0171 WRITELN (DEL H = DELTA 0 : 2)
0172 WRITELN
0173 WRITELN (Q = 4585 * (SQRT (DELTA) = Q 8 : 2)
0174 WRITELN
0175 WRITELN (VELOCITIES)
0176 WRITELN DESCRIPTION SMALLER BIGGER
0177 WRITELN
0178 WRITELN (DIA (m) 24, D1, 10 : 2, D2, 8 : 2)
0179 WRITELN (AREA (m.m) 24, A1, 10 : 2, A2 : 7 : 2)
0180 WRITELN (VELOCITY = Q/A (m/sec) : 24, V1 : 10 : 2, V2 : 8 : 2)
0181 WRITELN (SQU V)/2G (M) 24, M1, 9 : 3, m2 : 9 : 3)
0182 WRITELN
0183 WRITELN (B) CALCULATION OF THE CONSTANT K)
0184 WRITELN
0185 WRITELN (K FOR THE STRAIGHT PIPE OF SMALLER DIA : K1 : 5 : 2)
0186 WRITELN (K FOR THE STRAIGHT PIPE OF BIGGER DIA, K2 : 5 : 2)
0187 WRITE (K FOR THE GRADUAL EXPANSION OR CONTRACTION OF PIPE DIA)
0188 WRITELN (K3 : 5 : 2)
0189 WRITE (K FOR THE SUDDEN EXPANSION OR CONTRACTION OF PIPE DIA)
0190 WRITELN (K4 : 5 : 2)
0191 WRITELN (K FOR THE BENDS IN PIPE, KS)
0192 FOR I = 1 TO 6 DO)
0193 BEGIN
0194 WRITELN (I : 5 : KS : [I] 15 : 3)
0195 END
0196 WRITELN
0197 WRITELN
0198 WRITE
0199 WRITELN
0200 WRITE (0 1 2 3 4 5)
0201 WRITELN (6 7 8)
0202 WRITE
```

```
0203 WRITELN
0204 WRITE (NO D Z M H1 H2)
0205 WRITELN ( DELH TVAR[I] H = 3 + 4 + 7)
0206 WRITE
0207 WRITELN
0208 FOR I = 1 TO 37 DO
0209 BEGIN
0210 WRITE (2, I : 2, 3, DIA : 5 : 2, 4, Z [I] : 5 ; 2, 4 H[I] : 5 : 2)
0211 WRITE (4, H2 [I] : 5 : 2, 4, DELH [I] : 5 : 2, 3, TVAR [I] : 7 : 2)
0212 WRITELN (2, H[I] : 7 : 2)
0213 WRITE
0214 WRITELN
0215 END
0216 WRITELN
0217 WRITELN
0218 WRITELN (0 10 11 12 13)
0219 WRITELN
0220 WRITELN (SECT HL K L F = HL * K/L)
0221 WRITELN
0222 FOR i 1 TO 37 DO
0223 BEGIN
0224 WRITELN (1:2, 1 + 1 : 2, 3, HL [I] : 5 : 2, 5, K[I] : 5 : 2, : 5)
0225 WRITELN (D [I] 5 : 2, 4, F[I] : 0 ; 4)
0226 WRITELN
0227 END
0228 WRITELN
0229 WRITELN
0230 WRITELN (TOTAL ENERGY LOSS IN PIPE = SUM : 10 : 4)
0231 END
```

APPENDIX B
Preparation of reagents

1. Uniform acid concentrations

The following acid concentrations are recommended for general desk use : 6 N, 1 N, 0.1 N and 0.02 N. The preparation of these concentrations is presented in the following table.

Item	HCl	H₂SO₄	HNO₃
Specific gravity (20°/40°C)	1.174-1.189	1.834-1.836	1.409-1.418
Percent of active ingredient	36-37%	96-98%	69-70%
Normality of conc. reagent	11-12	0.36	15-16
Volume (ml) required to prepare 1 litre of			
18 N	—	500	—
6 N	500	167	380
1 N	83	28	64
0.1 N	8.3	2.8	6.4
Volume of 6 N to prepare 1 litre 0.1 N (ml)	17	17	17
Volume of 1 N required to prepare 1 litre 0.02 N (ml)	20	20	20

2. Uniform sodium hydroxide concentration

Prepare cautiously by dissolving the required amount (as in table below) in distilled water. Clarify the solution of sodium carbonate precipitate by keeping it at the boiling point for a few hours in a water bath or by letting the particles settle down.

Normality of NaOH solution	Required weight of NaOH to prepare 1 litre of solution	Required volume of 15 N to prepare a 1 litre of solution
15 N	625 gm	—
6 N	240 gm	400 ml
1 N	40 gm	67 ml
0.1 N	4 gm	6.7 ml

3. Methyl orange solution

Dissolve 500 mg of methyl orange powder in distilled water and dilute to 1000 ml.

4. Phenolphthalein solution

Aqueous : 5 gm of phenolphthalein disodium solution in distilled water and dilute to 500 ml.
Alcoholic : Dissolve 5 gm phenolphthalein in 500 ml 95% ethyl or isopropyl alcohol and add 500 ml of distilled water.

5. Erichrome black T

Mix 0.5 to 1.0 gm charcoal dye in 100 ml of ethylene glycol.

6. Potassium chromate indicator

Dissolve about 50 gm of neutral potassium chromate in a small quantity of distilled water. Add silver nitrate solution to produce a slight red precipitate. Allow to stand overnight and filter. Make up to 1 litre.

7. Acid-zirconyl-alizarin reagent

Dissolve 300 ml zirconyl chloride oxyhydrate, $ZrOCl_2 \cdot 2H_2O$ in 50 ml distilled water contained in a 1 litre glass stoppered volumetric flask. Dissolve 70 mg of 3-alizarin sulfonic acid sodium salt in 50 ml distilled water and pour slowly into zirconyl solution while stirring. This is the zirconyl-alizarin reagent.

Prepare mixed acid solution by diluting 101 ml conc. HCl to approx. 400 ml with distilled water. Carefully add 33.3 ml of conc. H_2SO_4 to 400 ml distilled water. After cooling, mix two acids.

To the zirconyl-alizarin reagent, add the acid solution and add water to 1 litre mark and mix. The reagent colour changes from red to yellow.

8. Alkali-iodide-azide reagent

Dissolve 500 gm NaOH (or 700 gm KOH) and 135 gm NaI (or 150 gm KI) in distilled water and dilute to 1 litre. To this solution add 10 gm sodium azide, NaH_3 dissolved in 40 ml distilled water. This reagent should not give a colour with starch solution when diluted and acidified.

9. Sodium thiosulphate, 0.1 N

Dissolve 25 gm $Na_2S_2O_3 \cdot 5H_2O$ and dilute to 1 litre with distilled water.

10. Standard silver nitrate titrant, 0.0141 N

Dissolve 2.395 gm $AgNO_3$ in distilled water and dilute to 1,000 ml. Standardise against 0.0141 N NaCl using potassium chromate indicator. Store in brown bottle. (1 ml of $AgNO_3$ is equal to 500 µg Cl.)

11. Standard sodium chloride, 0.0141 N

Dissolve 624.1 mg NaCl (dried at 14°C) in chloride free water and dilute to 1,000 ml. (1.00 ml = 500 µg Cl)

12. Standard fluoride solution

Dissolve 221.0 mg anhydrous sodium fluoride, NaF, in distilled water and dilute to 1,000 ml (1.00 ml = 100 µg F) to prepare stock solution. Dilute 100 ml stock solution to 1,000 ml with distilled water (1.00 ml = 10.0 µg F).

13. Buffer solution (for hardness test)

Dissolve 16.9 gm NH_4Cl in 143 ml of NH_4OH; add 1.25 gm of magnesium salt of EDTA and dilute to 250 ml of distilled water. This solution is also available commercially.

14. Standard EDTA titrant, 0.01 M

Weigh 3.723 gm of dry powder, dissolve in distilled water and dilute to 1,000 ml.

15. Manganese sulphate solution

Dissolve 480 gm $MnSO_4 \cdot 4H_2O$, 400 gm $MnSO_4 \cdot 2H_2O$ or 364 gm $MnSO_4 \cdot H_2O$ in distilled water, filter and dilute to 1 litre. The manganese sulphate solution should not give a colour with starch when added to an acidified solution of KI.

16. Starch solution

Prepare the aqueous solution by adding a cold water suspension of 5 gm arrowroot or soluble starch to approximately 800 ml of boiling water, with stirring. Dilute to 1 litre, allow to boil for few minutes, and let settle overnight. Use the clear supernate. This solution can be preserved with 1.25 gm salicylic acid per litre or by few drops of toluene.

17. Sodium thiosulphate stock solution 0.1 N

Dissolve 24.82 gm $Na_2S_2O_3 \cdot 5H_2O$ in boiled and cooled distilled water and dilute to 1 litre. Preserve by adding 5 ml chloroform or 1 gm NaOH per litre.

18. Standard sodium thiosulphate titrant, 0.025 N

Prepare either by diluting 250 ml sodium thiosulphate stock solution to 1,000 ml or by dissolving 6.205 gm of $Na_2S_2O_3 \cdot 5H_2O$ in fresh distilled water and diluting to 1,000 ml. Standard solution may be preserved by adding 5 ml chloroform or 0.4 gm NaOH per litre or 4 gm borax and 5-10 mg HgI_2 per litre.

19. Standard potassium dichromate solution 0.025 N

A solution equivalent to 0.025 sodium thiosulphate contains 1.226 gm/L $K_2Cr_2O_7$. The $K_2Cr_2O_7$ should be previously dried at 103°C for 2 hours.

20. Potassium fluoride solution (for D.O. test)

Dissolve 40 gm $KF \cdot 2H_2O$ in distilled water and dilute to 100 ml.

21. Phosphate buffer solution

Dissolve 8.5 gm potassium dihydrogen phosphate, KH_2PO_4, 21.75 gm dipotassium hydrogen phosphate, K_2HPO_4, 33.4 gm disodium hydrogen phosphate heptahydrate, $Na_2HPO_4 \cdot 7H_2O$ and 1.7 gm NH_4Cl in about 500 ml of distilled water and dilute to 1 litre.

22. Magnesium sulphate solution

Dissolve 22.5 gm $MgSO_4 \cdot 7H_2O$ in 1 litre of distilled water.

23. Calcium chloride solution

Dissolve 27.5 gm anhydrous $CaCl_2$ in distilled water and dilute to 1 litre.

24. Ferric chloride solution

Dissolve 0.25 gm $FeCl_3 \cdot 6H_2O$ in 1 litre of distilled water.

25. Standard potassium dichromate solution 0.25 N

Dissolve 12.259 gm $K_2Cr_2O_7$ in 1000 ml of distilled water.

26. Sulphuric acid reagent

Conc. H_2SO_4 containing 22 gm Ag_2SO_4 per 9 lb bottle (1 to 2 days required for dissolution).

27. Standard ferrous ammonium sulphate titrant, 0.10 N

Dissolve 39 gm $Fe(NH_4)_2(SO_4)_2 \cdot 6H_2O$ in distilled water. Add 20 ml conc. H_2SO_4, cool and dilute to 1000 ml. Standardize with standard $K_2Cr_2O_7$ daily.

28. Ferroin indicator solution

Dissolve 1.485 gm 1,10-phenoanthroline monohydrate, together with 695 mg $FeSO_4 \cdot 7H_2O$ in water and dilute to 100 ml.

APPENDIX C
Water Quality

Characteristics	Tolerance limit
1. Turbidity (JTU unit)	10
2. Temperature	25°C
3. Colour (pt-co scale)	20
4. pH	6.0-9.0
5. Solids (mg/L)	500-1500
6. Hardness ($CaCO_3$ scale) mg/L	200-600
7. Chlorides (mg/L) max	600
8. Fluorides (mg/L) max	1.5
9. Cyanides (mg/L) max	0.01
10. Selenium (mg/L) max	0.05
11. Lead (mg/L) max	0.1
12. Total chromium (mg/L) max	0.2
13. D.O. min.	40 percent saturation value or 3 mg/L whichever is higher
14. B.O.D. mg/L max	3.0
15. Phenolic compounds	0.005
16. α-activity μc/ml max	10^{-8}
17. Gross β-activity μc/ml max	10^{-8}
18. Oil and grease (mg/L) max	0.1
19. Coliform organisms monthly average, MPN/1000	Not more than 5000